CHANGE TO A POSITIVE MINDSET AND EXTEND YOUR LIFELINE

A JOURNEY TO MILES OF SMILES, POSITIVE ENERGY POWER, HOPE, HEALTH AND HAPPINESS

Edith Namm & Rita Kaufman

COVER DESIGN BY RITA KAUFMAN

authorHOUSE®

AuthorHouse™
1663 Liberty Drive
Bloomington, IN 47403
www.authorhouse.com
Phone: 1-800-839-8640

First published by AuthorHouse 8/31/2011

ISBN: 978-1-4634-4477-8 (sc)
ISBN: 978-1-4634-4476-1 (e)

Library of Congress Control Number: 2011913628

Printed in the United States of America

Any people depicted in stock imagery provided by Thinkstock are models,
and such images are being used for illustrative purposes only.
Certain stock imagery © Thinkstock.

This book is printed on acid-free paper.

**Dedicated to all
who have increased
our smile mileage in our journey
to
Positive Energy Power**

**"Give me a fish and I eat for a day.
Teach me to fish and I eat for a lifetime."
An old Chinese Proverb**

Dear Reader,

I am a Certified Specialized Handwriting Analyst, Counselor, Educator, and a thyroid, breast, colon and liver cancer survivor who has authored 6 books on stress management and is dedicated to sharing simple, safe, specific self-help strategies that can free your mind from fear and fill your mind with hope.

Change To A Positive Mindset And Extend Your Lifeline takes you on an exciting, unique journey to discover what it takes for you to feel self-confident, set realistic, achievable goals, and increase your smile mileage. You will discover:

- The "write way" to manage the stressful feelings of anger, anxiety, and sadness.
- The impact of emotional stress on all body systems.
- The winning ways to boost the Immune System.
- PEP (Positive Energy Power) Aerobics – the "write way" to feeling good from sunrise to sunset.
- PEP One-Liners that challenge negative thinking.
- Wise and witty words, and word game activities that have the power to positively activate the brain and body.
- The food/mood connection – The chemical/emotional energy connection.
- The color energy connection to your mood, food, clothes and environment.

Planning and preparing the road map for your journey to miles of smiles, positive energy power, hope, health and happiness has been an exciting and rewarding experience for me. I welcome you aboard. Travel at a speed that is comfortable for you. As Confucius said, "It does not matter how slowly you go, as long as you do not stop." Travel with the confidence of knowing that from the top of your head to the tip of your toes, you have learned to live a healthy lifestyle – one that can positively empower you to survive and thrive in a 24/7 stress-filled world.

Enjoy your journey to Positive Energy Power!!!. Wishing you miles of smiles, today, tomorrow, and always!!!

Edith Namm

Websites: www.enamm.com
           www.share-a-smile-ambassadors.com

A ROADMAP For CHANGE TO A POSITIVE MINDSET
A Guide to Inform, Encourage, and Support You Any Time of Day or Night

FOREWORD

POSITIVELY SPEAKING - UP FRONT AND CENTER

The words and issues on everyone's mind these days are "CHANGE", "HEALTH", and "ENERGY".

It is my goal to address the issues of "change", "health" and "energy" as they specifically relate to you and your ability to survive and thrive.

As you begin your <u>unique</u> journey to <u>change</u> your mindset, it is important to zero in on an understanding of the words "unique" and "change".

Basic Concepts To Keep In Mind:

Each human being is unique. Each one has his/her own unique features, bio-chemical profile, personality traits, experiences, beliefs, viewpoint, fingerprints, and handwriting style. No one is or can be exactly like anyone else.

You <u>only</u> have the power to change your own thoughts and actions. You have the power to change your relationship with food. You have the power to <u>choose</u> how you will react to people, events and situations.

There are internal and external dynamic changes taking place every second.

Nothing ever stays the same. No set of circumstances ever repeat themselves in the same identical way.

You are not what you were yesterday. You are what you are today. What you are today, will determine what you will be tomorrow.

It takes one moment to initiate a change that can affect the direction of your whole life.

The only time changes can be made is in the powerful present. Today is where the action is. Today's action forms the foundation for your future.

Change begins with what you choose to stop and what you choose to start.

Change begins with the words you choose to use and the words you choose to lose.

Change begins when you take the daily triple 'A' challenge – choosing what to adopt, adapt and apply in order to satisfy your specific needs.
Positive thinking creates change. Positive action makes things happen.
Positive thoughts and actions give you Positive Energy Power (PEP).

The tendency is to look on the outside for answers to problems. The bottom line is that the answers are to be found within you. Use the *Change Your Mindset* roadmap to show you the winning ways to get in touch with the answers that are waiting within you to be discovered.

IT IS WHAT IT IS

It is what it is – there are things you can't change
To be happy, it's your thinking you need to rearrange

Accept whatever is unjust or not right in your mind
Allowing you to embrace the peace you'll then find

When those in your world sadden or disappoint you
Forgive, let go and move on – it's the thing to do

Surround yourself with positivity day after day
For gladness and joy to be here and happily stay

Seek out people who think as positive as you
Those who feel enthusiastic and optimistic too

Enjoy friends, fun, relaxation and hobbies galore
And gratitude for the blessings that enrich you even more

Rita Kaufman

THE NEED TO CONTROL

Control is a word that's just seven letters long
But, oh, how it's possible to do you so wrong
It's something you may have to or need to be in
But its power takes over and you cannot win

You cannot control others - try as hard as you may
It only brings stress with each word you may say
It's their life, not yours – of that you can rely
It is what it is – something you cannot deny

People have choices, but it's theirs to make
People take chances, but it's theirs to take
What's good for you may not answer their need
And your advice, for sure, they will never heed

Control your frustration – pull in the rein
Leave others alone – try to refrain
Put a handle on this urge to control others so
Put all in perspective – self-talk till you know

You can control only you and your thoughts alone
Your beliefs, actions and reactions to set your own tone
Let others do the same – each family member and friend
Just be ready to listen with love – that's your message to send

Rita Kaufman

INTRODUCTION TO THE WORLD OF GRAPHOLOGY

GRAPHOLOGY TODAY

BASIC CONCEPTS of GRAPHOLOGY in a SIMPLIFIED CAPSULE FORM

BASELINES and 't-bars'

FASCINATING HANDWRITING FACTS

YOUR BRAIN – A POWERFUL PERSONAL COMPUTER

GRAPHOLOGY TODAY

In France, England, Germany, Switzerland, Holland, Canada, South America, and the United States, Handwriting Analysts are making significant contributions in the areas of Personnel Selection and Management Screening, Medicine, Psychiatry, Sociology, Criminology, Education, and Marriage/Compatibility Counseling.

In Courtrooms around the World, the testimony of Handwriting Experts is used to determine whether an individual is capable of committing a particular type of crime.

Graphology cannot determine an Individual's age, race, sex, or marital status.

Graphology can, however, serve as a reliable, unbiased, and non-judgmental tool to identify an Individual's personality strengths, thinking patterns, and emotional state of mind at the time the words are placed on the paper.

Throughout the world, it is common procedure for candidates seeking responsible positions to have their handwriting analyzed. Graphologists do the personnel screening for Lloyds of London. Noted in the Wall Street Journal, 9/3/85, a Paris executive recruiter stated that at least 80% of France's largest companies use the services of graphologists in hiring employees, especially for executive and professional positions.

Handwriting analysis is recognized by the Equal Employment Opportunity Commission as being a non-discriminatory practice because the analyst is unaware of race, creed, religion or sex of the person whose handwriting is being analyzed.

Diseases such as cardio-vascular disorders, Parkinson's Disease, epilepsy, arthritis, diabetes, cancer, alcoholism, drug abuse, anorexia, bulemia, and compulsive eating disorders contribute to a loss of nerve control over muscular coordination. These existing diseases can be identified in handwriting samples because handwriting is a neuro-muscular activity and pen pressure and letter formations are affected. By examining handwriting under a microscope, Alfred Kanfer, deceased noted graphologist at Strang Clinic, was able to detect the presence of cancer. In his 30 years of research, he achieved 70-80% accuracy in detecting the neuro-muscular deterioration in malignancy patients.

Within a short period of time, handwriting analysis can identify an Individual's emotional nature and his underlying problem core issues. Behavioral problems can be differentiated from learning disabilities. It is possible to determine how well an Individual is using his intelligence Graphology is being used in Israel as an auxilliary science of education. Teachers find it useful in detecting introversion in students. Israel trains its border guards in graphology in order to detect undesirables attempting to enter the country.

Banks, law enforcement agencies and attorneys benefit from the services of "examiners of Questioned Documents"--trained, qualified graphologists who determine the authenticity of handwriting and signatures on legal documents such as wills, contracts, and leases. Testimony of handwriting experts is used in trial cases to determine whether an Individual is capable of committing a particular type of crime.

Graphotherapy is the treatment, by highly qualified graphologists, of personality flaws through deliberately made changes in handwriting. It is a simple form of behavior modification. Undesirable negative tendencies can be stopped and positive characteristics successfully developed. It is particularly effective in dealing with children because their character is in the process of being formed. France originated graphotherapy and authorized its use for disturbed children. Graphology is indeed an exciting science that points the way to understanding, insight, growth and change.

BASIC CONCEPTS OF GRAPHOLOGY IN A SIMPLIFIED CAPSULE FORM

The Grapho-Trait Detectors that show and tell a writer's personality traits and emotional state of mind at the time the words are placed on the paper are:
Slant Letter Size Pressure   Baseline

THE HANDWRITING SLANT reflects a writer's temperament and emotional response to environment, people, and the future.

The Handwriting Slant can lean to the right, left, or stand straight up and down.

A moderate rightward slant shows and tells that the writer is an extrovert - outgoing, friendly, sociable, affectionate, future-oriented and eagerly anticipates events to come.

A vertical slant that stands straight up and down, shows and tells that the writer is level-headed, sensible, logical, realistic, reserved, independent, analytical, and focuses on issues in the present time.

A leftward slant shows and tells that the writer is an introvert, self-oriented, reserved, and withdraws from social interaction.

Note: Correcting or criticizing a writer's slant or letter size, interferes with an Individual's unique personality traits, stifles individuality, creativity, originality, and causes fear, anxiety, inhibition, insecurity, and <u>Low Self Esteem.</u>

One Size Does Not Fit All!

A writer's letter size can be large, moderate, or small.

A writer's letter size shows and tells how a writer relates to his/her environment and his/her capacity for concentration.

A large letter size shows and tells that the writer is extroverted, people and action oriented, outgoing, outspoken, and energetic, has a need to be noticed, seeks recognition and approval of others, is concerned with generalities rather than specifics, and is unwilling to concentrate on small details or be confined to a limited area of space.

A moderate letter size shows and tells that the writer is practical, realistic, reliable, adaptable, socially well-balanced, and has average ability to concentrate.

A small letter size shows and tells that the writer is introverted, modest, analytical, precise, attentive to details, not too communicative, has a high level of concentration, and concentrates on one thing at a time.

Interesting Note:

When you increase your concentration, your writing simultaneously becomes smaller.

When you are tired of writing, you lose your ability to concentrate, and your writing becomes larger.

PEN PRESSURE can determine a Writer's Level of Energy, Vitality and Determination.

How lightly or heavily a writer presses on a ball point pen, at the time of writing, reveals his/her vitality, will power, health and emotional intensity. Moderately heavy pressure, represented by firm, dark, thick pen strokes, shows and tells that the writer is energetic, ambitious, assertive, determined, has a retentive memory, and is in good physical health

Light pressure, represented by fine, thin, light, pen strokes, shows and tells that the writer is gentle, calm, passive, sensitive, impressionable, easily influenced, lacks physical energy, determination and confidence, resists commitments, easily forgets and forgives.

THE BASELINE shows and tells a writer's mood, and attitude in dealing with the events in his/her life.

The Baseline is the line formed when writing on a blank piece of paper.

The Baseline direction may go uphill, downhill, or remain level. You can identify a rising, descending or level Baseline direction, by following the direction of the 1st word to the last word on a line of writing, The Baseline direction can vary from line to line. Moods constantly fluctuate. The Baseline direction reflects mood changes.

A Level Baseline Direction shows and tells that the writer is reliable, realistic, even tempered, and level-headed.

A slightly Bouncy Baseline Direction shows and tells that the writer is flexible, lively, and is feeling happy.

An Ascending, Rising Baseline Direction shows and tells that the writer is feeling energetic, optimistic, enthusiastic, joyful, and ambitious.

A Descending, Downward Baseline Direction shows and tells that the writer may be feeling depressed, discouraged, disillusioned, fatigued, unhappy, or ill.

My goal is to make you aware of a simple, accurate graphic way to get in touch with your feelings every time you put your pen to paper. Therefore, the focus is on learning to see what the t-bars show and tell in your handwritten messages.

IT DOES MATTER HOW AND WHERE YOU CROSS YOUR T-BARS.

After each sample of writing, circle the **letter 't'** in each word.

Tally the direction of **'t-bars'** to see your level of positive energy power at the time you put your pen to paper. Tallying is done <u>after</u> all thoughts have been expressed. Concern about letter formation while you are writing, interferes with the flow of energy that your thoughts are creating.

Tally the # of short, evenly balanced **'t-bars'** that are on the **'t-stem'**.

Tally the # of long, evenly balanced **'t-bars'** that are on the **'t-stem'**.

Tally the # of **'t-bars'** that are high on the **'t-stem'**.

Tally the # of **'t-bars'** that are low on the **'t-stem'**.

Tally the # of **'t-bars'** that are to the left of the **'t-stem'**.

Tally the # of **'t-bars'** that are to the right of the **'t-stem'**.

WHAT THE 'T-BARS' SHOW AND TELL

'T-bars' that are long, strong, balanced and placed close to the top of the 't-stem' show and tell that the writer has self-confidence, high self-esteem, sets realistic, achievable goals and has the power to overcome everyday obstacles.

The number of 't-bars to the left of the 't-stem' show and tell the degree of procrastination and frustration the writer experienced at the time of writing.

The number of 't-bars' to the right of the 't-stem' show and tell how much anger the writer experienced at the time of writing.

IMPORTANT TO NOTE:

Each handwritten sample is a <u>unique</u> message revealing your energy pattern and emotional state of being.

No page of handwriting contains letter formations that are uniform or identical in shape.

Some variations in letter formations naturally occur and are expected.

I trust that what you 'learn to see' on your journey to self- empowerment, will become a fulfilling experience for you.

Fascinating Handwriting Facts

Regardless of the Writing Style that has been learned, each Individual develops his/her own unique Writing Style that is as identifiable as his/her fingerprints.

It has been noted that the chances of 2 Individuals having Identical Writing Patterns is one in 68 trillion.

Chemical sensitivities, allergies, drugs, alcohol, medications, illness, and fatigue can alter an Individual's Handwriting. Changes in Pressure, and in Letter Size and Shape, can be noted within 20 minutes after an allergic substance has entered the Body.

EMOTIONS AFFECT THE RHYTHM OF FINGER MUSCLE MOVEMENTS

Finger action is controlled by two sets of hand muscles -- the Extensors and the Flexors.

The Extensor Muscles extend the fingers to form upward strokes and rightward movements - rounded relaxed formations.

The Flexor Muscles contract the fingers to form downward strokes, leftward movements - straight and angular formations.

Steady rhythmic contraction and release movements across the page indicate the Extensors and the Flexors are operating in harmony with each other. There is a smooth, continuous flow of contraction and release movements. The writer is in harmony with self and surroundings.

Anger, Fear, and Anxiety disrupt rhythmic muscle functioning. The Flexors remain taut and tense and prevent the Extensors from making rounded relaxed formations. This causes angular, narrow letter formations, closely spaced words, crowded letters, overlapping lines of writing. The writer is feeling tense and irritable.

YOUR BRAIN --- A POWERFUL PERSONAL COMPUTER

Everyone is born with a Personal Computer that never sleeps -- a Brain. For your entire lifetime, your Brain is the processing center for all your thoughts, feelings, and experiences. All information concerning what you hear, see, smell, taste, and touch is stored in your Brain's Memory Data Bank.

Brain impulses direct all activity and movements. For the purpose of handwritten communication, your Brain retrieves information from its Memory Data Bank and in a fraction of a second, sends neuro-muscular impulses to your hand and fingers. The hand and fingers move the pen to record the feelings, thoughts and ideas that your Brain wishes to express. The hand is the neuro-muscular connection between the Brain and the paper. Handwriting is really Brainwriting!!!

Every handwritten message can show and tell a writer's inner feelings at the time the pen is applied to paper. I believe that handwritten communication is the "write" way to get in touch with the inner feelings of anger, fear, sadness, love, joy, and hope. It's the "write" way to safely relieve angry, sad, anxious feelings any time of day or night without the risk of personal confrontation or rejection. It's the "write" way to effectively increase your positive energy power (PEP) and experience the feelings of love, joy, hope, contentment, and fulfillment.

BOTTOM LINE
CHOOSE TO BE YOUR OWN BEST PEN PAL!!!

Equipment needed: a pen and your own helping hand
Materials needed:
> an unlined notebook for practicing PEP Aerobics
> an unlined notebook for PEP Journaling – recalling and recording daily happy experiences
> a supply of unlined <u>loose</u> sheets for The Ideal Way To Manage Emotional Stress – anger, fear, anxiety, and depression

INSIGHTS INTO THE FUNCTION OF THE MOST DYNAMIC, COMPLICATED, COMMUNICATION PROCESSING CENTER IN THE UNIVERSE

YOUR UNIQUE BRAIN

FOCUSING IN ON THE SENSORY/BRAIN CONNECTION

THE DESCRIPTIVE WORD CONNECTION TO A VIVID IMAGINATION

INSIGHTS INTO THE FUNCTION OF THE MOST DYNAMIC, COMPLICATED, COMMUNICATION PROCESSING CENTER IN THE UNIVERSE –– YOUR UNIQUE BRAIN

COMPLEX CONCEPTS SIMPLY STATED IN CAPSULE FORM

Structure of the Brain

The Brain is a part of the Central Nervous System and is located within the skull. The Cerebrum, the largest part of the Brain is divided into 2 hemispheres (right and left sections). Each hemisphere is divided into 4 lobes (regions): Frontal lobe, Parietal lobe, Occipital lobe, Temporal lobe. Each lobe has a specific function:

> The Frontal lobe is the portion of the Brain that manages memory, emotions, hearing, language and deals with intellectual tasks, decision making, goal setting, problem solving.
>
> The Parietal lobe is the portion of the Brain that receives, processes, coordinates and interprets sensory information about taste, smell, texture, and deals with motor skills and movement.
>
> The Occipital lobe is the portion of the Brain that controls vision, identifies colors, processes the words you see.
>
> The Temporal lobe is the portion of the Brain that manages memory, emotions, mood stability, music, sounds heard and processes into meaningful information words that are read and written.
>
>> The Hippocampus is involved in memory, learning and emotions. Its main function is in directing information to long term memory, taking incoming sensory information and packaging and processing the separate stimuli and sending them to the cortex where information becomes part of the long term memory.

The left Hemisphere deals with numbers, logic and rational thinking.
The right Hemisphere deals with abstract thinking, emotions, creativity, intuition and color.

The deep Limbic System – the emotional center, located near the center of the brain – sets the emotional tone of the mind. It stores highly charged emotional memories, controls appetite, sleep cycles and processes the sense of smell.

Fascinating Brain Facts

Each one's Brain is unique.

The Brain weighs 3 lbs. and is made up of a network of billions of neurons (brain cells). Each neuron has quadrillion connections to other cells in the body and is constantly busy receiving and sending electrical and chemical signals to your body organs, nerves, muscles and tissues. Information travels at the speed of 60 miles per hour.

From the first day to the last day of your life, the Brain receives, organizes and distributes all information that you see, hear, smell, taste, touch and experience. Your Brain is involved in every part of your life – all the thoughts, feelings and actions that take place every second in your entire lifetime. Your Brain is in charge of all your vital body functions. The Brain is 80% water and 30% oxygen and needs a daily supply of water, oxygen and nutrients to function efficiently. The Brain uses 20% of the body's blood flow and oxygen supply. Blood brings oxygen, glucose and nutrients to the Brain and takes away carbon dioxide and other toxic waste materials. Dehydration and a low level of oxygen can affect one's ability to think clearly and remember things.

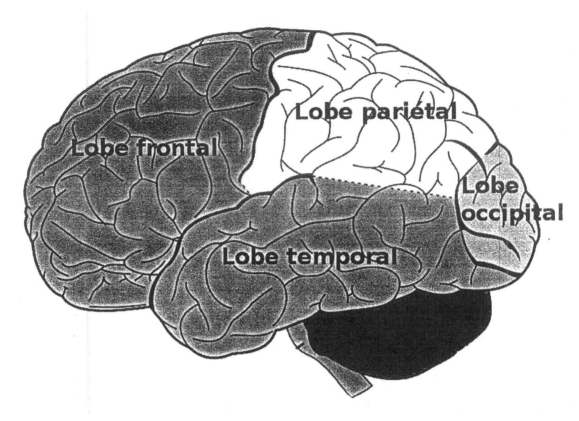

THE LOBES OF THE BRAIN

Essentials For a Healthy Brain and Body

Your body is composed of approximately 70% water. It is important to drink at least 4-6 glasses of water a day to prevent dehydration. Dehydration causes fatigue. Water transports nutrients throughout the body, maintains normal body temperature, cleanses all body systems and helps the kidneys remove toxic waste from the body.

Focus on deep breathing to adequately oxygenate your brain and body.

Sleep at least 6-8 hours for relaxed pleasant dreams.

Eat healthy foods.

Avoid toxic substances.

Your brain craves stimulation and thrives when it is being challenged. The brain responds to stimulation by adding more branches to the nerve cells and forming more connections. A daily dose of "r" activity will positively keep you calm, cool and connected. Read and reflect upon the PEP one-liners. Each day brings endless opportunities for new learning experiences. Recall and record your pleasurable learning experiences.

FOCUSING IN ON THE SENSORY/BRAIN CONNECTION

Facts about your sensors and your Sensory Nervous System

You learn about your surroundings through your sensors:

     what your eyes see – colors, shapes, objects, actions

     what your ears hear – words, sounds

     what your nose smells

     what your tongue tastes

     what your skin and hands touch

Your **Sensory Nervous System** is a network of billions of neurotransmitters (nerve cells) that are designed to transfer information about your unique sensory experiences to the brain in a fraction of a second.

Information about what your **eyes** see goes to the retina of the eye. The retina transmits the message to the optic nerve. The optic nerve carries the message to the brain. The brain interprets the image.

Sounds produced by pressure waves in the air cause your eardrums to vibrate. Vibrations are converted into signals that stimulate the thousands of auditory cells in the auditory nerve. The auditory nerve transmits signals to the brain. Neurons in the brain translate the signals into sounds.

Your **nose** has millions of smell receptors that can identify thousands of smells. Scent molecules enter your nose when you inhale air. The different structured molecules create different smells. Scent molecules stimulate your smell receptors. The receptors send signals to the olfactory nerve receptors. The olfactory nerve receptors send messages to the brain. It takes one sniff to stir your brain's memory and influence your behavior and mood. Certain smells can cause you to immediately salivate. The smell of chocolate can influence behavior and mood as early as in infancy.

Your **tongue** has thousands of taste buds. Each taste bud has a nerve connection that sends impulses to your brain. Your brain processes the information and determines if your food is salty, sour, sweet or bitter.

Your **skin**, palms of your hands and your fingertips have hundreds of thousands of receptors that are sensitive to pressure and temperature. Each fingertip is sensitive to the temperature, texture and pressure of any object that you touch or grasp. The skin surface of each fingertip has pores, nerve endings and ridges (Rugae Ridges) that detect temperature, texture and pressure beneath your skin and send signals to your brain. Your brain interprets the signals in terms of size, shape, texture and temperature. The index finger tip is the most sensitive of all your fingertips.

DID YOU KNOW?

A running nose is your body's attempt to flush out chemical sensitivities.

Tears contain a bacteria destroying antiseptic called Lysozyme that washes away toxic substances.

Saliva contains antiseptic chemicals that attack germs entering your mouth.

Coughs are your body's attempt to expel germs, fluids and irritating particles.

Chemicals that are absorbed through your skin, immediately permeate within your entire body.

A scratch or puncture of the skin provides the opportunity for germs to gain immediate entry into your body and cause possible infection It is important to wash your hands before eating, in order to cut down on germ entry.

THE DESCRIPTIVE WORD CONNECTION TO A VIVID IMAGINATION

Descriptive words have the power to create vivid images in your mind by stimulating those parts of the brain that are concerned with processing emotions, memory, language, words and sensory experiences.

The sound or meaning of a descriptive word can appeal to your sense of sight, hearing, taste, smell or touch.

Choose to use the **Descriptive Word List** to create vivid word pictures when recording what you see, hear, taste, smell and touch.

WORDS THAT APPEAL TO YOUR SENSE OF SIGHT

brilliant clear cloudy crinkled crooked crowded curved dark dim deep filthy flat fluffy foggy fuzzy gleaming glistening glowing hazy hollow high low misty muddy narrow pale round radiant shadowy shady shiny smoggy shallow steep sparkling spotless square stormy straight wide

Size
big bulky colossal enormous gigantic huge immense large little long miniature short small tall tiny

WORDS THAT APPEAL TO YOUR SENSE OF HEARING

banging beeping booming buzzing chirping clanging clattering clicking cracking crackling crashing creaking crunching dripping grinding groaning growling hissing honking humming hushed loud moaning murmuring noisy purring plopping quacking ripping roaring rustling screaming screeching shrill snarling splashing squeaking squealing squishing tinkling thumping thundering wailing whining whispering whistling

WORDS THAT APPEAL TO YOUR SENSE OF SMELL AND TASTE

bitter delicious fragrant juicy peppery ripe salty sour spicy sweet tangy tasty tasteless tart

WORDS THAT APPEAL TO YOUR SENSE OF TOUCH

bumpy cold cool cuddly damp dirty dry dusty frosty fuzzy gooey greasy grimy hard hot icy pointy prickly rough sharp slimy slushy smooth soft silky sticky wet wooden

BOTTOM LINE

BE AS BUSY AS A BUZZING BEE USING YOUR 5 SENSES – SIGHT, SOUND, SMELL, TASTE AND TOUCH – TO LEARN SOMETHING NEW EACH DAY.

A JOYFUL DAY AT THE BEACH

Sitting one day at the beach
I look all around just to see
So many wonderful sights
All freely available to me

A few birds chirping in flight
People in deep conversation
Ocean water and sand by my feet
Happily feeling the sensation

Shovels and pails of all sizes
Being filled by children with sand
Beach umbrellas from one end to the other
And parents with sun-block in hand

Children building castles nearby
All ages happily playing together
Older folks enjoying the sun
Relaxing in the beautiful weather

Adults walking the beach with friends
Some swimming in the ocean so blue
Little kids collecting shells to paint
And laughing at jokes that are new

People around me reading books
Others munching away
Surfers balancing on waves
Everyone enjoying their day

Energized by my feelings and thoughts
I enjoy this beautiful view
A sense of calmness returns
To my body, my mind and mood too

It's now time to leave the beach
Uplifted by this glorious day
Relaxed and ready to move on
With positive things going my way

Rita Kaufman

MOTHER NATURE'S GIFT

Eighty-eight degrees is what the prediction read
In actually, ninety-two is what the weatherman said

What a bonus! - usually out of reach for April weather
So we headed to the beach, the two of us together

An orange and green neon kite sailed over the sand
A dad and his daughter followed with string in each hand

The waves splashed happily as they hit the shore
With wondrous recollections of the summer before

People sat under umbrellas or on towels to relax
With not a thought of their problems, computers or fax

The sound of the ocean resonated so well
Like the beautiful ring of a perfectly pitched bell

It was a joyous time and from Mother Nature, a gift
As we smiled and enjoyed this well-deserved lift

We stayed in the moment and enjoyed each one
Then placed it in our Memory Bank and titled it fun!

Rita Kaufman

SPRING

My favorite is the season of spring
As beautiful as a butterfly's wing
Flowers in bloom for us all to see
A feast for the senses, so joyfully

Blue skies above and the day so bright
Pretty colors around that are just right
Mother Nature's gift - this special dress
A wonderful sight that's sure to impress

Folks all around us enjoying their mood
Everyone is smiling – no one is rude
Cheery and bright is the daylight sun
Bringing joy and happiness to everyone

Rita Kaufman

ENJOYING A NOVEMBER GIFT

Sitting on a bench overlooking the beach and the ocean
I see low fences in preparation for the cold winter ahead
But today is a beautiful Saturday in mid-November
And the chilly air is replaced by warming sunshine instead

The pavement, beach and playground are filled with people
From the very young to the elderly, all enjoying this day
Varied languages spoken representing different cultures
As they walk, run, play and sit, smiling and feeling okay

A few surfers glide upon the gentle waves of the ocean
Birds sunning themselves instead of taking their flight
Children riding bikes or happily having fun playing
Smiling, laughing, and enjoying their time with delight

I feel grateful for this gift from Mother Nature
Allowing us to shed the warm jackets once more
To share with others a hint of summer left behind
And add memories to the ones collected before

Rita Kaufman

RELAXING BY THE POOL

I sit by the pool in the warm Florida sun
Welcoming the rays, so relaxing and fun
The gentle bubbling of the Jacuzzi, I enjoy with a sigh
Along with the soft sound of the fountain nearby

I notice reflections within the pool as I glance
Palm trees move and sway a gentle dance
The Jacuzzi, fountain and reflections – all three
Bring a smile to my face and a calm stress-free me!

Rita Kaufman

SITTING BY THE BAY

Soft and rhythmic waves grace this sunny day
As I watch the calming water glistening on the bay
Swans gently swim, so beautifully at will
While boat after boat, stand silent and still

A nearby bench provides a place to sit and view
Sights and sounds, some old and some new
A little girl, cradled in her mother's arms so tight
Sees the beauty of nature in this wondrous sight

It's a place to listen to music or read
Or sit and relax to fill every calming need
Time appears to stop and worries seem to melt
And with it, serenity and peace can warmly be felt

The sun begins to set, and it's almost time to go
But the feeling of contentment continues to grow
The emotions that so beautifully touched this day
Will be etched in my memory and will always stay

Rita Kaufman

STAYING IN THE PRESENT

I quietly sit and observe things that are near
The things that I see and the sounds that I hear

I observe a man as he proudly walks by
He's dressed very nicely in a suit and a tie

I observe lines that form boxes below my feet on the ground
With little shapes embedded – some square and some round

I observe five birds flapping their wings as they go
All have bright orange beaks and fly by in a row

I observe floating clouds that are puffy and white
Creating unique formations that are quite a sight

I hear the bark of a cute little dog on a leash so long
His owner joyfully whistling an uplifting song

I hear the sound of a plane quickly passing in flight
And imagine passengers awaiting vacation delight

When I look and listen for things all around
I clearly realize with each sight and each sound

No racing thoughts of the past or future ahead
Now I'm right here in the present instead

Such observation spent in a most positive way
Lets you stay in the here and now each day

The present moment is the place to be
To focus and enjoy living life happily

Rita Kaufman

THE AWARENESS OF TREES

Slowly walking down the street
My eyes focus upon the trees
They gently swing and gently sway
As if they're dancing in the breeze

Their leaves slowly give way to change
On streets throughout the town
Beautiful, vibrant colors appear
Red, yellow, orange and brown

Some trees are light and delicate
Others are regal and strong
No matter how each one may look
Together, in a row, they all belong

Trees give us a place for shade
As they so beautifully grow
Take some time to look and see
You'll smile on each block you go

Rita Kaufman

WALKING DOWN THE AVENUE

I enthusiastically walked down the avenue today
Each street had its own flavor and so much to say
Delicious aromas of restaurants filled the air
With delightful sniffs of tasty culinary fare

Children perfecting moves in the Karate school
Masters guiding each child with a respectful rule
Clothes swishing around in the Laundromat
Machines and people going this way and that

Folks in offices filing and typing away
Reaching for coffee and cake from a tray
In the window of the beauty salon I could see
Women sporting their hairdos, as beautiful as can be

Banks busy with money going in and going out
Doing business with customers as they go about
Dental and medical offices available to help those
In need of assistance, from their head to their toes

A sad reminder of tough times so wrong
Many stores shut down way too long
Hopefully, the economy will improve once more
With hope and positive energy reopening each store

I'm thankful for so much going on each day
For stores and services; for places to go or stay
I'm grateful for this walk and the store owners so kind
For pleasant conversation and many smiles to find

Rita Kaufman

THINKING THROUGH THE SENSES

Think pleasant thoughts, especially before bed
Choose positive words to clear your head
Think of something to make you smile
Then repeat them as you relax for a while

Think of something nice that you <u>see</u> each day
Envision it in your mind's eye to make it stay
An enjoyable movie, family photo or a delicate tree
A painting or a child sitting upon your knee

Think of a <u>smell</u> that brings you joy and delight
To help you peacefully close your eyes at night
Morning coffee just brewed or a warm apple pie
A piping hot turkey or beautiful flowers nearby

Think of something that makes your <u>taste</u> buds soar
Then treat yourself to the memory even more
Spaghetti and meatballs or a delicious cake
Cookies, ice cream or hot soup to make

Think of something you <u>touch</u> that brings warmth inside
Something cozy or tender to remember with pride
A child's little hand or golden sand on the beach
Long silky hair or that special star you can reach

Think of the many sounds that you can happily <u>hear</u>
Things that bring delightful music to your ear
The rustling of crisp leaves or people laughing with joy
Your favorite songs or the cry of a newborn baby boy

Use your senses and the power of the five we own
Use them wisely and well to set a positive tone
Let them enrich your life from morning till night
And bring smiles to your face with energy just right.

Rita Kaufman

ROUTE 1 – EMOTIONAL STRESS/ PHYSICAL TENSION THE MIND/BODY CONNECTION

FOCUSING IN ON YOUR BUSY BODY SYSTEMS

THE IMPACT OF EMOTIONAL STRESS ON THE BODY SYSTEMS

FOCUSING IN ON YOUR BUSY BODY SYSTEMS
COMPLEX BASIC CONCEPTS - SIMPLY STATED

Your **Peripheral Nervous System** -- A network of billions of neurotransmitters -nerve cells - that electro-chemically communicate with one another in a fraction of a second.

Motor Neurotransmitters, upon messages received from your Brain, get your voluntary motor muscles to move -- walk, talk, sit, jump.

Sensory Neurotransmitters are designed to transfer information about your unique sensory experiences to your Brain. Every sensory experience changes the chemistry of every cell in your body. No two sensory experiences are ever duplicated.

Your **Autonomic Nervous System** monitors and regulates your automatic body functions - Digestion, Breathing, Heartbeat and Blood Pressure.

Your **Sympathetic Nervous System** stimulates your body systems in times of stress and danger. When one experiences emotional stress, it is the Sympathetic Nervous System that supplies the energy needed to handle short term emergencies. Chronic emotional stress results in chronic illness and inability to digest food and absorb the nutrients needed for the body to function. The mind and body fail to function effectively.

Your **Parasympathetic Nervous System** calms your body systems down after the emergency has passed and keeps your body systems functioning with optimum efficiency so that you can feel calm, cool and connected and enjoy good health.

Your **Endocrine System** regulates the functioning of your entire body and maintains your body's inner bio-chemical balance. The system controls your metabolism, growth, and circulation, helps your body deal with stress, regulates the secretion of all your hormones into your bloodstream.

Your **Adrenal Glands** (The Fight or Flight Glands) secrete more than 40 hormone chemicals that influence the mineral level in your Blood and in times of stress, release adrenalin, the stress hormone.

Your **Thyroid Gland** speeds up or slows down your body's metabolism rate for burning food for energy.

Your **Pituitary Gland** secretes hormones that stimulate the activity of all your body organs and glands and is responsible for your growth hormone.

SIGNIFICANT INTERACTION OF YOUR ENDOCRINE SYSTEM

If one gland does not function properly, other body parts will also malfunction.

Your **Respiratory System** is responsible for the oxidation process that takes place in your lungs - the exchange of oxygen and carbon dioxide.

Your **Cardio-Vascular Circulatory System** - Your Heart and your Blood Vessels - is responsible for the circulation of blood and oxygen to all your body cells.

Your **Heart** is responsible for automatically pumping your blood around to every cell in your body.

Your **Arterial Blood Vessels** distribute chemical nourishment to every cell in your body and contain antibodies to defend your body against attack, fibrinogen to stop hemorrhages, proteins (amino acids) needed for muscle, organ, and tissue repair, carbohydrates and fats needed for energy, minerals, hormones, and all glandular secretions.

Your **Venous Blood Vessels** carry the waste from every body cell and the excess water and debris from protein metabolism (carbon dioxide).

SIGNIFICANT INTERACTION

Your **emotions** affect the dilation or contraction of your small arteries, which affect your blood circulation and its chemistry. Inability for the blood to supply the required oxygen to your body cells, results in oxygen starvation. Physical symptoms of oxygen starvation may be weakness, fatigue, depression.

Your **Digestive System - Your Stomach, Liver, Gall Bladder, Pancreas, Small Intestine, Large Intestine** are concerned with the breakdown of your food into the simple chemical energy needed for every cell in your body.

Your **Stomach** manufactures the enzymes which chemically break down complex foods into simpler substances which can be absorbed into your bloodstream.

Your **Liver** regulates your sugar metabolism, stores glycogen (the energy from digested food), destroys and rids your body of bacterial poisons.

Your **Gall Bladder** releases the bile which breaks down fats so they can be picked up by the bloodstream and distributed to your body cells.

Your **Pancreas** secretes pancreatic juices to aid in the digestive process of sugars, starches, fats, and proteins and secretes insulin which promotes the utilization of sugar. Insufficient insulin distribution causes Diabetes.

Your **Small Intestine** absorbs the chemical nutrients from food.

Your **Large Intestine** provides the enzymes and hormones necessary for adequate digestion and eliminates the digestive wastes through the colon.

Your **Kidneys** maintain the acid-alkaline mineral balance in your body and dispose of toxic waste through the bladder in the form of urine.

Your **Immune System** -- An army of White Blood Cells (T-Cells and B-Cells) protect your body against infections from germs, bacteria, and viruses that gain entry into your body through the food you eat and the air you breathe.

SIGNIFICANT INTERACTION

Chronic stress and a deficiency of any nutrient can weaken your Immune System. A daily regimen of balanced, allergy-free, chemical-free, multi-vitamin and mineral supplements is your best assurance that your nutritional needs are being met. Especially helpful in maintaining a strong Immune System are Vitamins A, B-Complex, C, and E and the Minerals - Calcium, Magnesium, Selenium and Zinc.

Each Body System plays an important role in producing a total state of Well-Being.

Each Body System requires a chemically well-balanced nutritional program for optimum functioning.

THE IMPACT OF EMOTIONAL STRESS ON THE BODY SYSTEMS

Your mind continuously and automatically communicates with your body. Your body is designed to respond to all your feelings within a fraction of a second. When you experience stress to situations that anger, irritate, frighten, confuse, or endanger you, your Brain uses neurotransmitters as messengers to transmit this information to all your Body Systems.

Your Endocrine, Circulatory, and Immune Systems are alerted to respond to the stressful emergency.

Your Sympathetic Nervous System takes over. Your Adrenal Glands release adrenalin and cortisol into your bloodstream. Your Pituitary Gland releases powerful hormones that make your blood pressure soar. Sugar flows into your bloodstream for a quick burst of energy. There are chemical changes in the rate and intensity of the rhythmic functioning of your heart, lungs, and digestive tract. Your heart speeds up to pump the blood faster. Your lungs work faster and your breathing becomes rapid and shallow. Your blood flow, containing needed oxygen, is switched from your skin and digestive organs to your Brain and leg muscles. Your muscles contract and tighten up, causing increased muscle tension. Your digestive process slows down to let your body concentrate its energy on the stressful situation. Your mouth feels dry - saliva is not being used for digestion.

Consequences of Intense, Prolonged Stress on the Body Systems

A weak Immune System that lowers your body's resistance to disease.

An exhausted Endocrine System that overloads your body with stress hormones, creating hormonal imbalance and pain in vulnerable parts of your body.

An overworked Sympathetic Nervous System that can cause excessive muscle tension and pain in face, neck, chest, back, arms, and legs.

A Digestive System shut-down that interferes with food absorption, causing depletion of vitamins, minerals, and proteins that are essential for the formation of muscles, hormones, bones, brain, and nerve cells.

Sleep disturbances.

Fatigue and inability to concentrate.

Illnesses that are linked to intense, prolonged stress and tension are Allergies, Backaches, Diabetes, Digestive Disorders, Heart Disease, Hypertension, Respiratory Ailments, Skin Disorders, Tension Headaches.

LISTEN TO YOUR BODY SIGNALS

Your body is a wonderful complex structure with an amazing power to heal itself.

Your body needs your cooperation in order to function effectively and efficiently, 24/7.

Your body is constantly sending you signals.

Your body lets you know when it needs nutritional energy. The signal is a feeling of hunger.

Your body lets you know when it is time for sleep in order to repair and revitalize itself.

The signal is fatigue and drowsiness.

Your body lets you know when something is wrong - a chemical imbalance, a deficiency or weakness exists. The signal is pain and discomfort.

BOTTOM LINE

TAKE GOOD CARE OF THE ONE BODY THAT YOU HAVE FOR A LIFETIME!!!

ROUTE 2 – THE IDEAL WAY TO MANAGE EMOTIONAL STRESS

THOUGHTS TO KEEP IN MIND

YOUR MIND AND BODY NEED ENERGY TO FUNCTION

FOCUSING IN ON FEELINGS OF ANGER, SADNESS, DEPRESSION
AND ANXIETY

THE WRITE WAY TO TRAIN THE BRAIN TO DRAIN THE PAIN OF
ANGER, SADNESS,
FEAR AND ANXIETY

THE NEED FOR FORGIVENESS

THOUGHTS TO KEEP IN MIND

All your experiences – positive or negative- from the first day of life to the last – are processed by your Brain and stored in its Memory Data Bank as:

(+) The Positive Energy/Health Plan – PEP (POSITIVE ENERGY POWER)

                    or

(-) The Negative Energy/Health Plan – TNT (TOXIC NEGATIVE THINKING)

Looking into the benefits of the **PEP Plan**, we find:

> Feelings of love, hope and happiness
> An optimistic attitude
> Kind, winning words and friendly actions that have the power to make you feel good inside and out
> Satisfying relationships
> High self-esteem
> When you feel happy, your voice sounds light, lively, cheerful and soft.
> The corners of your mouth turn up to form a smile.

Looking into the risks of the **TNT Plan**, we find:

> Feelings of fear, anger and sadness – emotional stress
> A pessimistic attitude
> Unkind words and unfriendly actions that cause painful problems and fail to make you feel good inside and out
> Dysfunctional relationships
> Low self-esteem
> When you feel angry, sad or anxious, your voice sounds low, gloomy and cheerless.
> The corners of your mouth turn down to form a frown.

Either it's **PEP** or it's not. If it's not, it's **TNT. TNT** tends to keep one stuck in a rut and tied up in not's.

PEP generates stability, balance, moderation and consistency.

TNT generates instability, imbalance, extremes and inconsistency.

BOTTOM LINE

WHAT YOU THINK AND DO, DEPENDS ON YOU AND THE ENERGY PLAN YOU CHOOSE TO USE.

IMPORTANT TO KEEP IN MIND

Emotional Energy is contagious!!! To feel good, seek exposure to PEP people. You can recognize Pep people by their smile.

To feel calm, cool and connected:

    Think positive before you act.

    Practice balance and moderation in everything you do.

    "Accentuate the positive and latch on to the affirmative." (Johnny Mercer)

PEP
THE "KNOW" PROGRAM
3 Y'S – YES, YES, YES
HOPE
HAPPINESS
OPTIMISM
PEACE OF MIND
ENTHUSIASM

TNT
THE "NO" PROGRAM
3 NO'S – NO, NOT, NEVER
FEAR
ANGER
FRUSTRATION
ANXIETY
SADNESS

BOTTOM LINE

The PEP Program begins with the words – Yes, I can.
The TNT Program begins with the words – No, I can't.

FAITH, HOPE AND A POSITIVE THOUGHT

Faith, hope and a positive thought
Come from within and cannot be bought
They conquer the fear that lingers around
So feelings of calm and contentment can be found
They dissolve the anxiety that holds on so strong
For pleasurable peace to sing its sweet song
They squash the anger that burns so deep
Allowing beautiful days and peaceful sleep
How do we maximize this trio so grand
Begin with positive self-talk that's close at hand
Write down your worries and let them go free
And enhance your soul with powerful energy
Add invigorating beliefs and deep breaths each day
For joy and happiness to come your way
Live with faith, hope and a positive thought
They come from within and cannot be bought

Rita Kaufman

HARPY THOUGHTS

Positive words I eagerly find
To represent thoughts within my mind
I choose the ones that provide for me
Happiness and optimism so beautifully

Those thoughts – each and every one
That brings forth enthusiasm and fun
The words that tend to guide my day
In such a nice and unique way

Hope for peace and harmony for all
And kindness when the need shall call
Joy in the actions taken along the way
Listening to what each person has to say

Love and sincerity for family and friend
From day's beginning till day's end
Smiles to give and smiles to share
To show everyone how much you care

Rita Kaufman

YOUR MIND AND BODY NEED ENERGY TO FUNCTION

Feelings and thoughts provide the emotional energy for the mind.
Food provides the chemical energy for your body.

Feelings influence what you think. What you think influences what you believe. What you believe affects your attitude, your behavior and your relationship with yourself and others.

Feelings are to be respected. Feelings are <u>not</u> to be criticized, ridiculed, or judged to be right or wrong, good or bad, real or imagined, true or untrue.

Emotional energy can be either positive or negative. Positive and negative feelings do not occupy the same space in the same body at the same time.

When you feel love, you do not feel anger.
When you feel happy, you do not feel sad.
When you feel secure, you do not feel fear.
When you smile, you do not frown.
When you hug, you do not fight.
When you laugh, you do not cry.
When you compliment, you do not criticize.

The positive feelings of love, hope and happiness are activated in response to pleasurable, caring, nurturing experiences, and empower you to satisfy your needs and cope with the stress of everyday living in our continually changing environment.

The negative feelings of anger fear or sadness are activated in response to painful, traumatic experiences of abandonment, abuse (verbal, emotional, physical, or sexual), betrayal, deprivation, neglect, or rejection and deprive you of the power to function effectively. Rage, built-up unresolved anger, if not appropriately expressed in words, can result in anti-social behavior towards one's self and others – in the form of addictions, compulsions, obsessions, or violence.

Fear is anticipation of pain in the future. Sadness is the realization of loss or disappointment.

Unresolved anger, fear, or sadness must be identified and appropriately expressed before there can be a successful behavior change and resolution of emotional problems.

4 LETTER WORDS TO KEEP IN MIND
Free your mind from fear plus past pain.
Fill your mind with hope plus love.

BOTTOM LINE

FOR EVERY MINUTE YOU ARE ANGRY, YOU LOSE 60 SECONDS OF HAPPINESS.
Ralph Waldo Emerson (1803-1882)

MY THOUGHTS

My thoughts are all my own
They're made up in my mind
At times they're not so good
But are mostly the right kind

I have power to make my thoughts
Positive and enthusiastic you see
It's part of the freedom that I have
To give this precious gift to me

My thoughts are very special
I believe they make life real
They tell me how to act
They tell me how to feel

When I'm sad and feeling down
With thoughts that make me pout
I try to turn them all around
And cancel negativity out

Thoughts that make life bright
Are the ones that serve me well
Thumbs up to the ones that work
Like a perfectly sounding bell

Rita Kaufman

FROM SAD TO HAPPY AND GLAD

At times we have the feeling of happy
At times we have the feeling of sad
But certainly, between the two
It's better to have the feeling of glad

How can we rid the feeling of sadness
For sure, it doesn't suit us at all
What can we do to turn it around
To make happy and glad our call

We can seek enthusiasm, hope and inspiration
As a viable solution and positive view
To allow all the sadness to diminish
And make room for smiles and happiness too

Rita Kaufman

WHAT MAKES YOU GLAD

What makes you glad
What makes you smile
What stretches happiness
To more than a mile

Is it one thing for you
And another for me
Each of us is unique
And as different as can be

Is it a relaxing vacation
A good movie or show
Is it a party or celebration
Or fun with someone you know

Is it licking an ice cream cone
Or finding a nickel
Is it a new pair of shoes
Or a nice, juicy pickle

It really doesn't matter
That, for sure, is true
As long as happiness
Is in whatever you do

Enjoy what makes you glad
Take it all in with a smile
Make the most of each day
And you'll be happy all the while

Rita Kaufman

FOCUSING IN ON EMOTIONAL STRESS
FEELINGS OF ANGER, SADNESS, DEPRESSION AND ANXIETY

Anger is a natural emotion that is here to stay, never goes away, and can be experienced any time, any place, at any age. Anger comes in many forms, shapes, sizes, intensities - frustration, hostility, irritability, impatience, jealousy, hate, fury, greed, moodiness, procrastination, resentment, rage.

It is necessary that anger be identified, expressed appropriately, released and defused. If ignored, denied or buried, anger will fester and become toxic chronic anger.

Chronic repressed anger is hazardous to one's emotional and physical state of well–being.

It destroys Self- Esteem, adversely affects every relationship by interfering with a person's ability to trust and relate well with others. It keeps an individual stuck in the period of time when the painful experience occurred, perpetuates emotional pain and physical tension and retards emotional growth. Chronic repressed anger prevents an individual from achieving a satisfactory resolution to a problem. If not addressed, chronic repressed anger increases in intensity to explosive levels of violence against one's self and others.

RECOGNIZE THE SIGNS OF ANGER IN ACTION

ANGER causes individuals to

- abuse, accuse, annoy, argue, attack, avoid relevant issues.
- badger, belittle, blame, bully.
- complain, condemn, confuse, criticize.
- deceive, defy, demean, demand, devalue, discourage, distract, dominate, downgrade,
- deny reality, disregard and disrespect the rights of others, distort the truth.
- exploit, exaggerate.
- falsify facts, find fault, filibuster, focus on personality weaknesses of others.
- generalize and use stereotypes to classify others.
- harass, hate, humiliate.
- insult, ignore what is positive.

- judge others unjustly, jump to conclusions based upon false, inaccurate assumptions.
- label, lie.
- misconstrue facts, misinform. manipulate in an attempt to control others.
- nag, neglect the basic needs and concerns of self and others.
- obsess.
- procrastinate.
- quarrel.
- reject personal accountability and responsibility, resist change, ridicule.
- sabatoge, scapegoat.
- tease, threaten.
- use excuses to delay positive action.
- victimize and violate the safety of others.
- wage war with themselves and others.
- zealously over react.

THE WRITE WAY TO DEAL WITH ANGRY FEELINGS

Whenever you feel annoyed, frustrated, impatient, irritated, outraged, or resentful, <u>write a letter</u> to a person you would like to see or talk to.

State specifically - when, where, and what happened that caused you to feel the way you do. Use the word or words listed above that best describe your angry feelings.

I feel or felt _____ when_____

After writing your letter, **<u>tear it up and throw it away.</u>** You have gotten rid of your angry feelings and made room for good feelings and pleasant thoughts.

Never go to sleep feeling angry. Writing out your angry feelings before going to sleep is the write way to go for pleasant dreams. Regardless of the weather outside, you will rise and shine and be able to positively face the new day.

SADNESS

Sadness is a result of experiencing a loss of a person's love through traumatic circumstances,-- death, divorce, illness, violence or a loss of possessions because of catastrophic disasters beyond one's control. Each individual has his/her own time frame for expressing grief. Each individual has his/her own way of expressing grief. There is no right or wrong way to grieve. There are stages within the Grieving Process. It is important for each individual to work through each phase in order to complete the Grieving Process. An individual who gets stuck in any one phase, remains with a sad, angry, fearful memory.

The Process of Grieving is a learning experience -- learning new ways to live through loss and disappointment.

Phases of the Grieving Process
- Denial
    Feelings of shock, disbelief, and helplessness
- Anger
    Having to face the reality of the loss
- Bargaining
    Seeking explanations, rationalizing, attempting to undo the loss.
- Depression
    Sadness over the loss.
- Acceptance
    Willingness to confront the loss and accept the fact that life is different and that it is time to move on.

Grieving individuals need support PLUS CARE.

P L U S -- Patience, Love, Understanding, Security
C A R E -- Comfort, Attention, Reassurance, Encouragement

THE WRITE WAY TO RELIEVE SADNESS

Whenever you feel bored, confused, defeated, depressed, disappointed, discouraged, disgusted, downhearted, exhausted, hopeless, helpless, lonely or unloved, <u>write a letter</u> to a person you would like to see or talk to.

Write about all the things that are making you feel sad. Use the word or words listed above that best describe your feelings and state specifically - when, where, and what happened that caused you to feel that way.

Your letter does not need to be mailed or kept. The letter has served its purpose. You have released your sad feelings and made room for good feelings and pleasant thoughts.

THE WRITE WAY TO TRIUMPH OVER TRAGEDY

Celebrate the **<u>Life</u>** of departed loved ones. Create a Memory Journal of joyful, humorous recollections to tell and pictures to show.

OUR TARKY

Many challenges unveil themselves day by day
But they make you stronger, or so they say
Some spur you to action that lasts for years
Others are emotionally charged and bring forth tears

Today's challenge, so emotional and sad
Our Tarky, laying quietly – his health so bad
We knelt down beside him and stroked his face
His tail weakly wagged with a gentle grace

We continued to pet him with tears streaming down
As he lifted his head to us with love surround
We think of the joy that Tarky always brought
To hold and cherish, for it can never be bought

While in the hospital we prayed he'd pull through
We were optimistic but there was little we could do
Thankfully Tarky returned to his home and family
Happy and grateful, but he was not the same we could see

We gave him undivided attention and love day by day
And each moment with him was a precious gift we would say
A few months later Tarky, getting weaker and ill
Left us for good and was now sadly still

But we hold on to the memories of our beloved furry friend
Who appreciated and loved us unconditionally till the end
We think of him with love through our tears
And celebrate the joy he brought through the years

His excitement at seeing us when we came close to the door
His wagging tail and kisses we knew were always in store
His closeness, cuddling and unconditional love so warm
Melted the stress and anxiety that challenged each storm

The walks with Papa that were loved by each
His loyalty to his family most humans don't reach
We think of how he looked into our eyes so strong
And know that together we all closely belong

He's woven into the thread of our family and forever will
We think of him with love and devotion whether busy or still
His endearing and playful spirit will never depart
Our Tarky will always have a place in our heart

Rita Kaufman

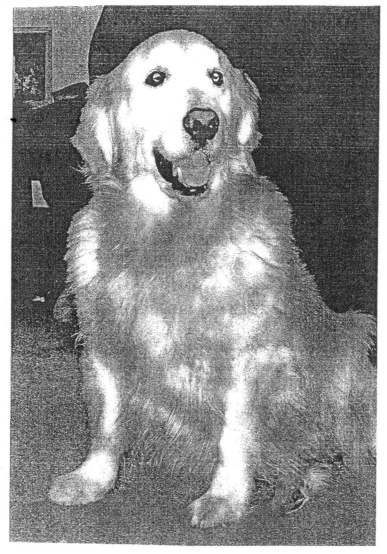

TARKY

THE MANY SIDES AND SIGNS OF DEPRESSION

DEPRESSION can be a reaction to an upsetting event or loss, an individual's inability to accept what is, or an individual's inability to appropriately express painful feelings. Depression can have varying degrees of intensity and duration. It can be mild, moderate, severe, transitory, or persistent in nature. Depression can affect any individual regardless of age, gender, or economic background. Depression can be the result of a change in family structure - divorce, death, illness, a loss of someone or something that has been loved or chemical changes within the body. A depressed person feels hopeless, helpless, and worthless and engages in self-destructive, risk taking, abusive behavior.

Depression Can Lead To Suicide.

Suicide is a cry for help to be noticed, an attempt to end the pain of depression, a self-destructive message that may be verbal or written.

CAUSES

A sudden loss of an important relationship.

Fear of Rejection.

Fear of Failure -- inability to live up to unrealistic expectations.

BEHAVIORAL CLUES

Inability to cope with the routine tasks of daily living.

Withdrawal from family, friends, and activities.

Giving away favorite possessions.

Increased use of drugs and/or alcohol.

Inability to concentrate, confused irrational thinking.

Loss of appetite.

Sleep disturbances.

Not goal oriented.

ALL SUICIDE THREATS - EXPRESSED VERBALLY OR IN WRITING -- MUST BE TAKEN SERIOUSLY!!!

Suicide threats are not to be denied, belittled or minimized. If you fear that someone is suicidal, never leave that person alone. Seek immediate professional help. Contact a Crisis Center.

GRAPHO-INDICATORS CAN SHOW AND TELL DEPRESSION OR SUICIDAL INTENT.
A COMBINATION OF INDICATORS MUST BE PRESENT TO HAVE AN ACCURATE ASSESSMENT OF DEPRESSION.

Illegible, tangled script, distorted letter formations.

Descending, erratic Baseline - words or word endings that droop below the Baseline.

Weak, poorly formed "t-bars".

NOTE:

Suicidal people usually kill themselves on impulse.

A Suicidal Baseline may involve only a few lines or words on a page of writing. A descent may suddenly appear in the last word or words, or last letters of a word at the end of a line at the right margin.

Studies have indicated that people who had successfully committed suicide tended to write short suicide notes.

Those who were unsuccessful in their suicide attempts, wrote long notes and managed to be saved in time.

ANXIETY

Anxiety exists when a situation, based upon the unknown, is viewed by a person to be a threat to his/her state of well-being. Anxiety is based upon fear of anticipated pain in the future -- "what if's" that are to be. An anxious person turns specific issues and situations into self-defeating generalizations, exaggerates their meaning and imagines the worst scenarios. Anxiety is based on inaccurate assumptions, distorted perceptions, misinformation, rumors, gossip or hearsay.

If ignored, denied, or buried, anxiety will fester and become toxic chronic anxiety.

THE WRITE WAY TO HELP WORRY, DOUBT AND FEAR TO DISAPPEAR

Worry, Doubt, and Fear about future events usually causes one to ask "what if?"

What if he or she doesn't like me?" "What if I make a mistake?"

Whenever you feel anxious, frightened, nervous, terrified, uptight, or worried about any future event, <u>WRITE A WASTE LIST</u> - A Worried, Anxious, Stressful, Tense Emotion list.

List all the "what if's" you are afraid will happen.

"What if _____

_____

"What if _____

_____

Now, change the words **"What if"** to **"Even if"** and then complete the thought with positive words.

"What if I were to make a mistake?" becomes "Even if I were to make a mistake, I'm still okay. I am not a failure.

"Even if _____ were to happen, I can handle it, because I choose to believe that I have the inner strength and power to deal with whatever happens.

State at least 2 steps you can take to handle each "what if" situation.

Even   if   _____   I   can

_____

Even   if   _____   I   can

_____

You'll find that by focusing on writing your "even if" statements, the present worry and fear will be relieved. Refer to the waste list a month later, you'll most likely find that many of your "what ifs" never happened. It's impossible to predict the future. It's important to deal with one day at a time.

BOTTOM LINE

BELIEVING THAT YOU CAN DEAL WITH WHATEVER HAPPENS, IS THE KEY TO FEELING CONFIDENT, COMFORTABLE AND SECURE.

The Write Way to Provide Positive Closure to Negative Statements

Use the antonym connection word "but".

"but" joins 2 thoughts together.

The second thought contradicts the first thought.

When writing statements that express worry, uncertainty, anxiety, pessimism, fear, discouragement or hopelessness, add any of the following positively energized words to complete your statement.

but I'll do my best.

but I can handle it.

but I can do it.

but it will be okay.

but I can get through it.

    but I will work it out.

Examples:

I feel discouraged <u>but</u> I will work it out.

I feel sad <u>but</u> I can get through it.

BOTTOM LINE

THE WORDS THAT FOLLOW THE WORD "BUT" CAN FREE YOUR MIND FROM FEAR AND FILL YOUR MIND WITH HOPE.

AN "I CAN DO IT" ATTITUDE INCREASES ONE'S LEVEL OF SELF-CONFIDENCE.

When you want doubt and fear to disappear, say the words, "I can do it! Yes! Yes! Yes!" at least five times. Increase your voice volume each time you say the words.

Raise your arms in mid-air and smile.

Your positive energy power (PEP) is reinforced by the height of your arm movement and the broadness of your smile.

BOTTOM LINE

SELF-CONFIDENCE GROWS EACH TIME A CHALLENGE IS MET AND INNER FEARS ARE OVERCOME!!!

LIGHT UP YOUR LIFE

Start <u>A Smile File</u>. List your favorite words, thoughts and enjoyable activities. Refer to the list when you want worry, doubt and fear to disappear.

WORRY

Worry is toxic – it's filled with negativity and more
Worry gets LOUDER, and for happiness shuts its door
Worry affects thoughts, feelings and behavior indeed
It grows WILD and STRONG, like a most unwanted seed

Worry gets you to a nasty, ugly and stressful place
With its sadness and anxiety, both so difficult to erase
It digs you into a hole – hard to climb out of, and then deepens in tone
It exaggerates feelings and thoughts and takes on a life of its own

How can we eradicate it? What can we do?
How do we deal with it so that we no longer feel blue?
Take deep breaths - in for four, hold for seven and out for eight
To relax us, calm us, and slow a rapidly climbing heart rate

Write about the negativity, the anxiety and the fear
The worry, the people or situations that bring forth each tear
Then rip up the paper in as many pieces as you need
To erase stress and calm nerves for a more relaxed life to lead

We can realize that worry does nothing at all to solve
Any problems, feelings or thoughts we need to resolve
So heed the above suggestions and put them into play
For a much brighter, happier and a smile-filled day

Rita Kaufman

THE MOUNTAIN OF LIFE

The mountain of life is overwhelmingly high
Fear and stress build as you anxiously try
How do you climb it - you question and ask
In your mind you ponder this difficult task

Stress and anxiety can take over your life
And can be as harmful as the cut of a knife
Whatever the concern, you need to find
A dependable solution to ease your mind

Taking baby steps you can readily see
Each one can be met, that is the key
Every step climbed is accomplishment felt
And with courage, the step ahead can be dealt

Anxiety will decrease and motivation will soar
The mountain to climb will appear easier than before
Make a list of these steps and put them in place
As one by one, you apply them with a smile on your face

Rita Kaufman

"Holding on to anger is like holding on to a hot coal with the intent of throwing it at someone else; you are the one who gets burned." --- Buddha

THE NEED FOR FORGIVENESS

Forgiveness is the key for successful survival - the first step for relieving emotional stress and restoring physiological balance to your body systems. Forgiveness is <u>not</u> about accepting, condoning, or agreeing with what caused you past pain. Forgiveness is about ceasing to blame or to feel resentment towards anyone for painful experiences suffered in the past. Forgiveness is about letting go of sad memories. Forgiveness is about giving yourself permission to get on with your life. Forgiveness is about coming to terms with what happened and taking positive action to heal, change, and move on.

BOTTOM LINE

FORGIVENESS CANCELS OUT ANGER AND GUILT AND MAKES ROOM FOR LOVE, JOY AND HOPE.

IN ORDER TO GROW, YOU NEED TO LET THE GRUDGES GO

Compile a Resentment List. Include the names of all persons towards whom you feel resentment for past painful experiences.

Write a letter to each person on your **Resentment List**. Tell when and where the past painful experience took place. End your letter with the following Forgiveness Statement:

I now choose to forgive you for all past painful experiences.

<u>The letter does not require mailing.</u> The letter serves as the "write way" to release the feeling of resentment that is living within you. To avoid any resentment build-up, constantly monitor the initial stroke of all words.

If you detect the presence of the resentment stroke, address the pain the "write" way, right away.

BOTTOM LINE

IT IS NECESSARY TO GET IN TOUCH WITH YOUR FEELINGS AND THOUGHTS IN ORDER TO CHANGE YOUR ATTITUDE, BEHAVIOR AND RELATIONSHIPS.

ROUTE 3 – PEP AEROBICS – THE WRITE, READ, SAY WAY TO FEEL GOOD FROM SUNRISE TO SUNSET

WHAT ARE YOU THINKING?

THOUGHTS TO KEEP IN MIND ABOUT THE POWER OF WORDS

TIME TO RETIRE THE BELIEF "PRACTICE MAKES PERFECT"

AN IDEAL MESSAGE TO KEEP IN MIND

WHAT A DIFFERENCE A PREFIX MAKES

WORDS HAVE THE POWER TO HURT OR HEAL

COMPLIMENTS EACH DAY KEEP THE INSULTS AWAY

A RIDDLE TO THINK ABOUT

WINNING WORDS FOR POSITIVELY ENERGIZED SELF-TALK

THE KEY TO A POSITIVE SELF-IMAGE AND SUCCESSFUL SOCIAL RELATIONSHIPS

THE WRITE WAY TO A POSITIVE SELF IMAGE AND BELIEF SYSTEM

POINTER-CISE

TO GO FROM MOPE TO COPE TO HOPE

THE ABC'S FOR POSITIVE THOUGHTS AND ACTION

WHAT ARE YOU THINKING?

Next to each statement listed below, put the number that reflects your thought pattern.

    1 point = rare thought

    2 points = frequent thought

    3 points = constant thought

_____ 1. I can't help myself.

_____ 2. I am a winner.

_____ 3. That's just the way I am.

_____ 4. I am proud of myself.

_____ 5. There's nothing I can do about it.

_____ 6. I am capable of doing anything I choose to do.

_____ 7. I'm not good at anything.

_____ 8. I am capable of learning anything I choose.

_____ 9. It's not fair.

_____ 10. I am honest, sincere, and open in my thoughts and opinions.

_____ 11. It's not my fault.

_____ 12. I am intelligent.

_____ 13. I never get a break.

_____ 14. I am responsible for my reactions, responses, and choices in my life.

_____ 15. It's not my day.

_____ 16. I am my own person.

_____ 17. I can't do it.

_____ 18. I am willing to change.

_____ 19. I don't like the way I look.

_____ 20. I am a good listener.

_____ 21. Trouble always follows me.

_____ 22. I am unique.

_____ 23. I'm a born loser.

_____ 24. I accept other people as they are.

_____ 25. Life is miserable.

_____ 26. I appreciate all that I do.

_____ 27. Whatever can go wrong, will go wrong.

_____ 28. I believe in myself.

_____ 29. I'll never see the light of day.

_____ 30. I choose to get things done promptly.

_____ 31. I worry about everything.
_____ 32. I choose to live happily.
_____ 33. I'm never lucky enough to win.
_____ 34. I am an optimist.
_____ 35. I'll think about it tomorrow.
_____ 36. I deserve to succeed.
_____ 37. If I wish hard enough and long enough, maybe it'll happen.
_____ 38. I do the best I can do in every situation.
_____ 39. I don't want to talk about it.
_____ 40. I find positive qualities in myself every day.
_____ 41. Everything I do, turns out wrong.
_____ 42. I have hope.
_____ 43. It'll never happen.
_____ 44. I have confidence in myself to solve my problems.
_____ 45. I'll never get over it.
_____ 46. I have will power.
_____ 47. I'll never forgive them for what they did to me.
_____ 48. I like who I am.
_____ 49. I'm always right.
_____ 50. I set goals and achieve them.
_____ 51. I can't be bothered.
_____ 52. I smile a lot.
_____ 53. I'm not good at making decisions.
_____ 54. I take responsibility for my actions.
_____ 55. I'm not interested in anything you have to say.
_____ 56. I believe that everything will turn out okay in the end.

Total the points of all odd numbered statements. _____

Total the points of all even numbered statements. _____

Which score is higher?
A higher score on odd numbered statements indicates a negatively energized thought pattern.
A higher score on even numbered statements indicates a positively energized thought pattern.

Choose to maintain positively energized thoughts no matter what happens. Your positive thoughts empower you to get through stressful times.

REPHRASING CAN POSITIVELY MAKE A DIFFERENCE.
Zero in to statements 1,7,15,17,19,43,45,47,53.
If the statement was rated 1,2 or 3, delete the negative word "no", "not", "never".
Enter the rephrased statement into your PEP workbook. Write each rephrased statement 3 times for 30 consecutive days.

BOTTOM LINE

REDUCE THE NUMBER OF TIMES YOU USE THE WORDS "NO", "NOT", "NEVER", AND YOU INCREASE YOUR PEP!!!
POSITIVE ENERGY POWER EMPOWERS YOU TO SUCCESSFULLY DEAL WITH DAILY OCCURRENCES OF NEGATIVE PAIN AND PREVENTS TOXIC NEGATIVE OVERLOAD. YES!!! YES!!! YES!!!

THOUGHTS TO KEEP IN MIND ABOUT THE POWER OF WORDS

The words you choose to use express your feelings and your thoughts. What you think affects what you believe. What you believe affects your attitude. Your attitude influences how you act. How you act influences your relationships with others.

Words generate positive or negative emotional energy. Positively energized words produce positive messages and are stored in the Brain's Memory Data Bank under the PEP Plan. Positive messages instill confidence, hope, enthusiasm, success and high self-esteem.

Negatively charged words provide negative messages and are stored in the Brain's Memory Data Bank under the TNT Plan. Negative messages instill fear, anger, anxiety, failure and low self-esteem.

It takes one word – positive or negative -- a fraction of a second to affect your emotional state of well-being and bio-chemically change your heart rate, blood pressure, breathing and digestion.

Words have the power to hurt and wage war. Words have the power to heal and win peace. Words have the power to unite or divide. It never hurts to say a kind word because a kind word never hurts.

BOTTOM LINE

CHANGE BEGINS WITH THE WORDS YOU CHOOSE TO USE AND THE WORDS YOU CHOOSE TO LOSE.

CHOOSE TO INCREASE AND STRENGTHEN YOUR POSITIVELY ENERGIZED WORD POWER AND BECOME AN IDEAL PEP COMMUNICATOR.

RX FOR A POSITIVELY ENERGIZED LIFESTYLE
A DAILY DOSE OF CPR CAN EMPOWER YOU TO STRIVE, THRIVE AND SURVIVE:

COMMITMENT + CONSISTENCY
PATIENCE + PRACTICE
REPETITION + REINFORCEMENT

THE WORDS WITHIN

Words are all around us
Words are within us too
Words can be delightful
Or change our point of view

The words that are within us
The ones that talk to us alone
Can be soft and mild in nature
Or loud and strong in tone

Our words can make us happy
Empower us with joy and delight
Or take us down in spirit
Hampering our day and night

We have the strength and power
To make the choice that's best
The many words that are spoken
Can stress our mind or let it rest

Words within can lead us
To places safe and secure
Words can encourage actions
That for anxiety is a cure

The words we choose are ours
Our thoughts allow this choice
Make them encouraging and hopeful
And let our body and soul rejoice

Rita Kaufman

TIME TO RETIRE THE BELIEF THAT "PRACTICE MAKES PERFECT".

Demanding perfection is an exercise in futility. The consequences are unrealistic expectations, disappointment, frustration and failure because of trying to reach an unobtainable goal.

BOTTOM LINE

ADOPT THE BELIEF THAT "PRACTICE MAKES BETTER". PRACTICE BALANCE and MODERATION IN EVERYTHING YOU DO.

TIME TO RETIRE THE OVERUSE OF THE WORD "PERFECT".

To accurately describe your feelings about a person, place, object or event, choose to adopt the words listed below:

> awesome appropriate best exact excellent exquisite fantastic great ideal magnificent marvelous masterful miraculous outstanding precise remarkable sensational splendid super supreme terrific wonderful

If greater descriptive emphasis is needed, it's okay to include any of the following words – one at a time:

> absolutely totally thoroughly positively

AN IDEAL PEP MESSAGE TO KEEP IN MIND

To increase your PEP, adopt the positively energized word "ideal" whenever you are tempted to use the word "perfect". The procedure is completely safe and non-toxic. There is no danger of overdosing.

What the positively energized word "ideal" tells you:

I   Improvement begins with I. If it is to be, it is up to me.

Id   Your Inner Dialogue puts you in touch with your unique needs.

Idea   Positively energized ideas empower you to achieve what is uniquely ideal for your comfort.

I deal effectively with the daily stress of living in an ever changing hectic world.

BOTTOM LINE
I STRIVE, I THRIVE, I SURVIVE!!! YES, YES, YES!!!

WHAT A DIFFERENCE A PREFIX MAKES!!!

A prefix is a syllable that is placed before a word. The prefix changes the meaning of that word. The syllables "in", "un", are prefixes that mean "not". When these prefixes are placed before a word, that word has a negative meaning.

INSTANT REPHRASING - REPLACING NEGATIVE WORDS WITH POSITIVE WORDS

Rx-For those individuals suffering from Positive Word Deprivation caused by chronic, intense, toxic Negative Word Overload

Treatment Procedure

Consult your Dictionary to perform an immediate word transfusion to increase your PEP vocabulary. There is a positive word for every negative word. Replace existing negative vocabulary words with their antonyms. Seek synonyms for positive words. Enter positive words into a PEP Word Journal.

For words that are positively not "in", drop the prefix "in" and the words are in to win.

inattentive	attentive
inconsistent	consistent
inappropriate	appropriate
incapable	capable
incompetent	competent
insecure	secure
insincere	sincere
intolerant	tolerant

Words that are "in" and give you power

Information   initiative   interest   introspection

Words that you can positively undo by dropping the negative prefix "un"

unaccountable	accountable
unaware	aware
uncaring	caring
uncertain	certain
uncomfortable	comfortable
uncomunicative	communicative
undesirable	desirable
undisciplined	disciplined
unfriendly	friendly
unhealthy	healthy
uninformed	informed
unrealistic	realistic
unsatisfactory	satisfactory
unsure	sure
untimely	timely
unwilling	willing

A "un" word that does well for you - understanding

Prognosis

Immediate increase in positive energy. Procedure is completely safe and non-toxic There is no danger of overdosing.

Sticks and stones can break one's bones
But words can hurt much more than stones.

WORDS HAVE THE POWER TO HURT OR HEAL

Cruel, uncomplimentary words damage an individual's self esteem. Those who experience uncontrollable anger or fear, use the tongue as a weapon to verbally attack and provoke anger and fear in others. This kind of attack is referred to as Verbal Abuse.

The words used for verbal attack tend to be inaccurate and uncomplimentary. They tend to be names and descriptive labels that criticize, demean, discredit, ridicule, insult, and humiliate an individual's abilities, appearance, or physical build. Some commonly used labels are: stupid, dumb, moron, idiot, fool, crazy, lazy, clumsy, miserable, selfish, failure, ugly, fat, slob.

Ridicule makes one feel inadequate, unworthy and uncomfortable. Teasing about issues over which one has no control, destroys one's self-confidence, breeds anger, frustration and resentment. Unfavorable comparisons create feelings of inferiority and self-doubt.

Repeated use of cruel words is a destructive, no-win means of communication. The person sending the negative message does not feel good. The person receiving the negative message does not feel good.

Make a list of any hurtful words you frequently use. Supply the antonym for each word and you have an instant positive word vocabulary available for you to use.

The way to prevent anger and resentment build-up when exposed to a verbal abuse attack is to write, read, and say to yourself the following statements as often as necessary. The words will serve as a successful defense strategy to block the effects of the verbal attack.

> I cannot control the thoughts or actions of others. I can control how I respond to others.
>
> I do not take the attack personally. When I take the angry words of others personally, I become emotionally involved and get caught up in their anger and lose sight of my ability to focus on relevant issues.
>
> It is not about me. I am not the cause of the problem. I have nothing to do with it.
>
> The inaccurate, untrue words are the expressions of an angry, insecure individual.

BOTTOM LINE
WE ARE NOT ON THE SAME PAGE.

COMPLIMENTS EACH DAY KEEP THE INSULTS AWAY

Positively energized words focus on one's unique strengths, talents and abilities, and celebrate what is attempted and achieved.

Compliments have the power to send self-esteem soaring.

Choose words from **Smiling From A to Z**, to fill in the blanks below:

I believe that you are _____.

I believe that I am _____.

SMILING FROM A to Z

A -- agreeable, affectionate, alert, ambitious, amiable

B -- beautiful, brave, bright, brilliant

C -- capable, caring, charming, cheerful, clever, competent, congenial, conscientious, considerate

D -- dedicated, delightful, determined, dynamic

E -- eager, empathetic, energetic, enthusiastic

F -- faithful, flexible, forgiving, friendly

G -- generous, gentle, giving

H -- happy, helpful, healthy, humane

I -- intelligent, interesting

J -- jolly, jubilant, just

K -- kind, knowledgeable

L -- lively, lovable, loyal

M -- marvelous, mild-mannered

N -- neat, neighborly, noble

O -- optimistic, outstanding

P -- patient, peaceful, polite, proud

Q -- quiet, quotable

R -- relaxed, reliable, respectful, responsible

S -- sensitive, sincere, strong, successful

T -- talented, thoughtful, trustworthy, truthful

U -- understanding, unique, unselfish

V -- victorious, vigorous, vivacious

W -- willing, wise, wonderful

Y -- young, youthful

Z -- zestful

CREATE PEP NAME PROFILES

Write the letters of a person's name in a vertical line.

Use SMILING FROM A TO Z to select one or more adjectives that begin with each letter in the name.

Send PEP Name Profiles to your favorite persons, including yourself.

BOTTOM LINE

KIND <u>HANDWRITTEN</u> WORDS CAN POSITIVELY CHANGE YOUR LIFE AND YOUR RELATIONSHIP WITH YOUR SELF AND OTHERS.

THE POWER OF WORDS

Words are heard and spoken as part of a given day
They communicate and fulfill us in a unique way
Words are used to heal us and they are used to calm
Words can excite us and words can cause us harm

There are many available words to choose
Positive ones to keep or negative ones to lose
But always remember to keep in mind
Let them be complimentary, pleasant and kind

Carefully choose the words to say or write
That will result in peace and not a fight
Choose among them all the while
Ones that bring forth a great big smile

Words have power; they can be sweet or strong
Select the ones that fit and appropriately belong
Both the speaker and the listener will feel just the same
The relationship will be smooth and happiness will remain

Rita Kaufman

THOUGHTS, WORDS AND ACTIVITIES

Try to make your thoughts and words
Sound pleasant, positive and kind
Choose only the ones that fit the bill
And leave the negative ones behind

The thoughts that come into your mind
And the words you choose to say
All combine to play a role
That bring forth a happy day

Select activities and hobbies
To enhance your joy and pleasure
Dance, draw or play a sport
For happiness to treasure

Strengthen your enthusiasm
Your effort and energy too
It's something that's so worthwhile
To inspire everything else you do

Rita Kaufman

A RIDDLE TO THINK ABOUT

What is at the root of all your beliefs and attitudes?

What reflects your experiences and your feelings?

What determines how well you function and survive?

What is active from the first moment to the last moment of your Life?

What can change from moment to moment?

What never sleeps or rests?

What has the power to heal or hurt?

What is unique for every individual?

What can make you feel comfortable, self-fulfilled, bring joy and peace into your Life?

What can provide the strength, courage, and willpower you need to successfully achieve your goals?

What can safely see you through difficult times?

What can make your day -- every day?

Answer to the riddle: Your Unique Internal Thoughts!!! (IT)

BOTTOM LINE
IF "IT" IS TO BE, IT IS UP TO ME!!!

KEEP "IT" SIMPLE!!!

S	SAFE
I	INVIGORATING
M	MODERATE
P	POSITIVE
L	LIKEABLE
E	ENLIGHTENING

WINNING WORDS FOR POSITIVELY ENERGIZED SELF-TALK

<u>Now</u> is the <u>time</u> to <u>choose</u> to positively energize what <u>"IT"</u> is.

<u>"IT"</u> is your <u>IV</u> (Inner Voice), <u>ID</u> (Inner Dialogue), <u>ST</u> (Self-Talk)

Self-Talk is based upon what you think and believe about yourself. We talk to ourselves 24/7. Self-Talk is like a continuous tape recording of words. It is important to become aware of the words that are being recorded into our memory data bank.

Each day, choose to read *The Winning Words for Positively Energized Self-Talk:*

> I accept and appreciate myself for who I am.
> I appreciate all the good things that I can do.
> I appreciate, respect and value my unique talents and abilities.
> I believe I have the courage and inner strength to get through difficult times.
> I believe I am an important individual.
> I believe I am a good and deserving person.
> I believe I have the power to solve my problems.
> I believe I have the ability to achieve anything that I make up my mind to do.

To reinforce your **Positive Self-Talk** messages, <u>say</u> *The Winning Words* in front of a mirror. Smile. Nod your head up and down. Avoid any side-to-side motion. End each thought with the words, "yes, yes, yes!!!" and a "thumbs up" signal.

Ideal time for reading *The Winning Words* is at sunrise and sunset.

BOTTOM LINE

YOU ARE WHO YOU THINK AND BELIEVE YOU ARE!!!

"No one can make you feel inferior without your consent" --- Eleanor Roosevelt

PEP THOUGHTS TO KEEP IN MIND

Self-esteem is not based upon heredity, intelligence, education, wealth, or social standing.

Self-esteem is based upon the amount of Positive Energy you generate, and your level of self-satisfaction and self-confidence.

When you spend your time and energy identifying and satisfying your unique specific needs, you are self- fulfilled.

Self-confidence grows each time a challenge is met and inner fears are overcome. Self-confidence supplies the energy and encouragement to move forward. Self-esteem sags when you are experiencing anger, sadness or fear. Self-esteem soars when you are experiencing happiness.

LIVING WITH POSITIVE ENERGY

Life goes on for us day after day
But how do we see it – what is <u>your</u> view
Is the glass half full or half empty
What strategies are useful for you

Life is a range of many challenges
Filled with hills and valleys that come to mind
Looking for signs of hope and optimism
Leaving pessimism and sadness behind

People look all around for answers
They look everywhere for clues to find
Spending days upon days of precious energy
But the answer is always in your own mind

It's the same world outside for others
But how <u>you</u> alone perceive it is key
Rid yourself of negativity, fear and anger
Keep your outlook as positive as can be

For inspiration and motivation to soar
Positive self-talk is the place to begin
Hope and enthusiasm will guide and lead you
And your self- esteem will enable you to win

Live your life filled with wonderful experiences
Send fear, anger, resentment and hatred away
Nothing is perfect, but can always be better
Love, hope and optimism can be here to stay

Make your actions and behavior productive
Breathe effectively and deeply each day
Compliment yourself as well as others
Make kindness your goal and your way

Smiles and laughter will be yours to enjoy
Success and satisfaction will be yours to hold
Your world will be confident and filled with happiness
As you embrace these strategies in the life that you mold

Rita Kaufman

SATISFACTION

What is the meaning of satisfaction
I know it's a feeling so good
How do you get it or find it
I'd like it to be understood

Satisfaction can be felt in many ways
From friends, chosen careers and wise decisions
From vacations, children, husbands and wives
And dreams realized from their original visions

Satisfaction may be felt from a word or a smile
From a wave or a pat on the back
From a vote of confidence given to someone
Whose self-esteem they sadly may lack

It may be found in the action you take
To make little things better each day
For family, friends or even a stranger
In a small, but significant way

So treasure the spirit of satisfaction
And the joy of fulfillment from the start
Be grateful as you interact with others
And feel the warmth of it inside your heart

Rita Kaufman

THE KEY TO A POSITIVE SELF-IMAGE AND SUCCESSFUL SOCIAL RELATIONSHIPS

The Key to a Positive Self-Image begins with having a satisfying relationship with yourself.

You need to accept and appreciate yourself before you can accept others.

You need to feel love for yourself before you can give love to others.

You need to be kind to yourself before you can be kind to others.

You need to feel respect for yourself before you can respect others.

You need to understand yourself before you can begin to understand others.

You need to value yourself before you can value others.

BOTTOM LINE

A POSITIVE SELF-IMAGE EMPOWERS YOU TO BE A POSITIVE ROLE MODEL AND TO RELATE EFFECTIVELY WITH OTHERS.

THE WRITE WAY TO A POSITIVE SELF-IMAGE AND BELIEF SYSTEM

A Positively Energized Self-Image and Belief System empowers you to form healthy relationships and successfully cope with the realities of life and function effectively in challenging situations.

DO YOU KNOW

The Personal Pronoun "I" is the only one letter word that represents the One most important Individual in the world.

The Personal Pronoun "I" is the only Pronoun that is always capitalized. Capital letters are always used to signify importance.

BE THE "I" YOU WANT TO BE

You are what you think.	I think, I am a winner!
You believe what you think.	I believe, I am a winner!
You are what you believe.	I am a winner!

From *A List of Positively Energized Words*, choose 5 positively energized adjectives that describe the "I" you want to be.

For each word selected, complete the following 3 statements.

I think, I am _____.

I believe, I am _____.

I am _____.

Write each set of 3 statements, 3 times each, every day for at least 30 consecutive days. It takes at least 30 consecutive days to successfully program your positive thoughts into your Memory Data Bank.

After 30 consecutive days, select another 5 positively energized adjectives and repeat the programming process. There is no limit to the number of adjectives that you may wish to include in your positively energized Belief System. Continue to increase the number of words so that the writing exercise lasts for 20/30 minutes.

After each writing session, check to see what your **'t-bars'** show and tell.

REINFORCE YOUR POSITIVE BELIEFS

Read and say your "I" statements in front of a mirror.

Smile. Nod your head up and down. Avoid any side-to-side motion.

End each statement in an animated way -- with a "thumbs up" signal.

Note your facial expression and tone of voice as you repeat your statements.

BOTTOM LINE

READ AND SAY YOUR "I" STATEMENTS TO YOURSELF ANY TIME YOU WANT TO FEEL GOOD ABOUT YOURSELF.

IT SUITS ME TO A "t" – A LIST OF POSITIVELY ENERGIZED WORDS

adaptable	attentive	adventurous	benevolent
comfortable	confident	conscientious	considerate
charitable	consistent	contented	cooperative
courteous	determined	devoted	discreet
effective	empathetic	energetic	enlightened
enthusiastic	faithful	good-natured	healthy
honest	hospitable	independent	individualistic
inquisitive	interested	inventive	lenient
mature	moderate	motivated	non-judgmental

nurturing	optimistic	patient	pleasant
practical	rational	realistic	receptive
respectful	satisfied	strong	sympathetic
tactful	tolerant	tranquil	trustworthy
understanding	versatile	victorious	worthy

Use Color Energy to Reinforce Your Belief System.

Complete the following "I" statements by selecting a trait listed below. Use the color pen suggested for the trait selected.

I think, I am _____.

I believe, I am _____.

I am _____.

USE ORANGE INK FOR
courageous
sociable
constructive
confident
willing

USE BLUE INK FOR
reliable
accepting
flexible
tranquil
trusting

USE YELLOW INK FOR
reasonable
logical
optimistic
articulate
forgiving
happy
organized

USE TURQUOISE INK FOR
calm
changing
triumphant
certain

USE GREEN INK FOR	USE PINK INK FOR
balanced	kind
efficient	supportive
methodical	considerate
appreciative	compassionate
secure	loving
contented	sincere
relaxed	

USE PURPLE INK FOR	USE RED INK FOR
proud	strong
open-minded	determined
worthy	energetic
accepting	

Reinforce your Positive Self-Image

Say your "I" Statements in front of a mirror.

Smile.

Nod your head up and down. Avoid any side-to-side motion.

End each statement in an animated way -- with a "thumbs up" signal.

POINTER - CISE

A simple exercise routine that is guaranteed to generate physical and emotional fitness, flexibility, balance, and self-esteem.

Who?

Positively recommended for everyone - regardless of age or gender.

When?

Number and length of daily sessions depends upon your need throughout each day.

Rhythm, speed and time devoted to Pointer-cising, is your decision.

Where?

Pointer-cising can be done in a standing, sitting, or reclining position. Your comfort is the determining factor.

What equipment is needed?

Your favored Pointer Finger, of either your right or left hand.

Physical examination is not required prior to Pointer-cising. There are no physical restrictions, limitations, side effects, or risks.

Pointer-cising Routine

1. Choose any "I" statement..
2. Bend your elbow and face the palm side of your hand.
3. Straighten your Pointer Finger. Relax all other fingers.
4. Your straight Pointer represents the word "I".
5. Bend your Pointer Finger and point to yourself as you say the remaining words in the statement.
6. Return Pointer to a straight position at the end of the statement.

Choose to say as many statements as many times as you wish.
Repeat steps 1 - 6 each time you read a statement.

Rationale for Pointer-cising

It focuses in on your own unique, individual concerns and needs.
It generates positive energy, action, and change.
It strengthens your inner power to be responsible and in control of your thoughts and feelings.
It allows you to recognize that resolution and power is found within.

Recommendations for added fun, pleasure, and animation when Pointer-cising
Draw a smile on your Pointer. (2 dots and a curve)
Place a Smile Sticker on your Pointer.

Warning:

<u>Never</u> use the Pointer in an outward direction. That destructive, fault-finding, blaming motion aims to hurt and results in anger, frustration, hate, negative emotional stagnation and depleted Positive Energy Power!!!!
Pointer-cise, Pointer-cise, Pointer-cise and you will Positively Energize!!!
Yes!!! Yes!!! Yes!!!

TO GO FROM MOPE TO COPE TO HOPE: PEP MESSAGES TO WRITE, READ, AND SAY ANY TIME OF NIGHT OR DAY.

Direction Words, when used in Idiomatic Expressions, can reflect positive messages. The words -- above, ahead, forward, in, on, toward, up -- reflect positive words and actions.

I am above board with myself and with others.

I rise above the problem to seek solutions.

I am ahead when I am on top of the situation.

I keep moving on to get ahead.

I look forward to each new day.

I can come up from under.

I always keep my hopes up.

No matter what circumstances I am in, I can come through it and get out of it.

It is up to me to empower myself.

I lean towards enjoying life.

I am up to changing to a positive way of life.

I am on the "up and up" with myself.

I am up to writing up what is up in my life.

BOTTOM LINE

ONWARD AND UPWARD IS THE WAY TO GO TO INCREASE YOUR PEP. THE SKY IS THE LIMIT!!!

PRACTICE THE A B C'S FOR POSITIVE ACTION

Assume responsibility for strengthening your Positive Belief System.
Believe that you can successfully handle anything that comes your way, and you have the key to feeling comfortable and secure.

Challenge yourself to discover alternatives. There are always options and alternatives to every situation.

Choose to spend your time and energy being involved in productive winning strategies.

Clarify what is confusing by dealing with one issue at a time.

Detoxify what is toxic.

Enjoy and treasure each pleasurable moment.

Focus on what you can do, not on what you can't do.

Focus on what brings self-satisfaction. Self-satisfaction builds Self-esteem.

Fortify what is vulnerable.

Glorify Life, Love, and Laughter.

Identify which feelings are at the root of your problems.

Justify what is valid.

Like what you have, rather than lament over what you do not have.

Modify what is extreme. Moderation is the key to a healthy mind and body.

Nullify what is negative.

Pacify what is turbulent.

Rectify what is unbalanced.

Recognize and appreciate your own importance and value.

Satisfy your unique individual needs -- safely and appropriately.

Seek facts to find solutions. Seek answers to "what, when, where, how".

Simplify Life by breaking down what is complex into simple manageable steps.

Verify what are assumptions, inaccuracies, or speculations.

Zero in on your unique and special talents and abilities.

BOTTOM LINE

POSITIVE THINKING CREATES CHANGE. POSITIVE ACTION MAKES THINGS HAPPEN.
POSITIVE THOUGHTS AND ACTIONS GIVE YOU POSITIVE ENERGY POWER!!!

A POSITIVE VIEW OF LIFE

Look at the smile and not at the pain
Think of the sunshine and not of the rain
Picture colors beautiful and bright
See the essence of life in the brightest light

Focus on the good and not on the bad
Concentrate on the glad and not on the sad
Follow your goals and each desired dream
Be positive, no matter how difficult they seem

Look at the inner beauty so strong within you
Your mind and your spirit in all that you do
Take pride in the accomplishments you've collected
Take equal pride in the many choices you've selected

Be encouraged, enthusiastic and hopeful each day
Free yourself from anger, fear and sadness in every way
Enable the presence of joy and welcome good news
Surround yourself with people who share these views

Be true to yourself and respectful of others
Friends, mothers, fathers, sisters and brothers
Let forgiveness and kindness rule each day
And peace and happiness will find its way

Rita Kaufman

REACH OUT

Reach out to family members
Reach out to your many friends
Embrace their help and support
And to you, this message sends

You're valued and very important
Unique and special, indeed
Your family, friends and self-talk
Will satisfy and nourish each need

Tell yourself that you are a winner
Believe what you say and it will serve
To give you the needed confidence
And help you when life throws a curve

Reach out to the skills that will help you
The strategies that guide you each day
Reach out for advice when you choose to
Your joy and happiness will soar in that way

Rita Kaufman

ROUTE 4 – THE IDEAL WAY TO PREP FOR PEP

THE WRITE RELIEF FOR A STRESSFUL POOR MEMORY

START EACH DAY THE PEP PLAN WAY

WISH TO DO TIME

THE WRITE WAY TO PREPARE FOR A GOOD NIGHT'S REST AND PLEASANT DREAMS

IT'S 1, 2, 3 TO BE THE BEST YOU CAN BE

1. Ready to adopt the PEP Lifestyle to satisfy your unique, specific needs.
2. Set your mind to write, read and recite your favorite PEP one-liners each day.
3. Good to go, grow, glow and grin!!!

THE WRITE RELIEF FOR A STRESSFUL POOR MEMORY

Create a simple organized system of Smiling Reminders for remembering dates, appointments, and scheduled activities.

1. Place pen and yellow pads near the phone and television set.
2. Write lists, lists, and more lists. Place smiling face stickers on top of each list.
3. Write a list of medications and supplements.
4. Keep shopping lists.
5. Write a list of names and phone numbers of important people and services.
6. Write a list of scheduled appointments to be kept.

CPR TO IMPLEMENT SOS for SPM (Stressful Poor Memory)

C -- commitment, consistency

P -- patience, practice, persistence

R -- repetitious reinforcement

To have peace of mind and effectively meet challenging situations, take your Power Kit with you when you leave home. Your PK includes your lists, pen and paper.

START EACH DAY THE PEP PLAN WAY

List all the things that you need to do.

List the fun activities you would love to do.

Simplify the list by giving priority to essential, urgent items. Consider the time, location and physical energy required to realistically accomplish the listed items. Include time for fun and relaxation to enjoy whatever pleases and interests you. At the end of the day, check off all you did and record your accomplishments in your joyful journal.

BOTTOM LINE

PLAN FOR BALANCE AND MODERATION IN EVERYTHING YOU DO!!!

A BALANCE OF FUN AND ROUTINE

Most of our days are like most of our days
They just flow and go in routine
But isn't it nice to have a day here and there
That's more special, exciting or serene

A fun outing or a day spent with friends
An overnight stay or a carnival ride
A Broadway show for you to enjoy
Things that make you feel happy inside

Sprinkling your life with fun and delight
Raises the bar for each ongoing day
Ideas of the moment or those happily planned
Balance daily routines in a wonderful way.

Rita Kaufman

"Wish To Do" Time

What would increase your smile mileage?

What would you love to do but until now you haven't given yourself permission to pursue?

Now is the time to live your dream.

Now is the time to make time for fun and happiness.

Now is the time to write a list of your hopes and wishes – things you wish to do, see, taste, learn, experience, explore, and achieve.

Sentence starters for each Wish Statement:

I wish to _____

_____.

When finished, prioritize your list.

Have fun establishing your priorities and determining which wish to act upon.

Check out the direction of the baseline of each statement.

Check out which "wish statement" has the greatest number of long, strong, balanced t-bars that are close to the top of the t-stem.

Monitor your smile mileage. Review your daily fun time schedule and record what you did to have fun that day.

BOTTOM LINE

TODAY IS WHERE THE ACTION IS. START TODAY TO MAKE YOUR DREAMS AND WISHES COME TRUE!!! CELEBRATE AND REWARD YOURSELF WHENEVER YOU HAVE FULFILLED A WISH!!!

STRESS RELIEF THE "WRITE" WAY

Choose topics to write about – anything under the sun
Let the words flow for stress relief and hours of fun

Write about something that makes you smile
Whatever comes to mind – it will take just a while

Select random acts of kindness aimed at a few
Or those from others that were given to you

Write about someone you admire so much
It will bring pleasure and keep you in touch

Think about something relaxing you like to do
Dancing, painting or knitting – hobbies old or new

Write about your family's shining star
A grandchild or friend that stands out by far

Make up an imaginative and funny story
For smiles and laughter to reduce your worry

Write about something you've learned or discovered
About the world or yourself that you've uncovered

Choose ideas from above or from those in your mind
Write them down and feel joy of the very best kind

Rita Kaufman

FAVORITE THINGS

Sun shining through windows as we awake
Put smiles on our faces to joyfully take
Funny jokes and stories to hear and to tell
Provide laughs each day for keeping us well

Kisses, hugs and gifts we generously share
Show friends and family how deeply we care
A helping hand and listening ear to lend
Being there for others with love to send

Friends to be with - a good meal to eat
Together make a most enjoyable treat
The laughter of grandkids that keep us young
Tickles, games played and songs happily sung

Computers, shopping and crafts to do
Sharing great ideas, both old and new
Good books, concerts and Broadway shows
Entertain us from our heads way down to our toes

Family recipes, photos and memories galore
Vacations with loved ones and so much more
Our favorite things energize a happy feeling
Keep us positive and enhance our healing

If I may suggest, here's something to do
It's been helping me and, hopefully, help you
Make a list of your favorite things and enjoy them so
And notice how quickly your smiles will grow

Rita Kaufman

HOBBIES

A hobby is something fun to do
It's quite exciting for me and you

Painting, dancing or a game of ball
Singing, chess or going to the mall

Puzzles, books, cards or knitting
Movies, talk shows or babysitting

Golf, music or games with words
Gardening, fishing or watching birds

Whatever you choose, it will entertain
In the sunshine or at home in the rain

A hobby makes you feel good inside
And for your emotions, it's a positive ride

Select one today, or maybe a few
It's guaranteed to bring smiles to you

Rita Kaufman

THE WRITE WAY TO PREPARE FOR A GOOD NIGHT'S REST AND PLEASANT DREAMS

Your brain and body need at least 7 to 9 hours of sleep each night. Sleep rejuvenates the brain. Less than 6 hours a night affects one's health and one's work performance, decreases the blood flow to the brain and interferes with one's ability to think clearly during the day. Never go to sleep feeling stressed. Write about any angry or anxious concerns you are feeling. When finished, **tear up your comments.** They are not to be kept or shared. You have gotten rid of your stressful feelings and made room for good feelings and pleasant thoughts.

Recall and record the good happenings that caused you to smile on this day. It's the "write way" for the body and mind to relax, rest comfortably and recharge itself with positive energy.

Regardless of the weather outside, you will rise and shine and be able to positively face the new day.

BOTTOM LINE

THE BETTER YOU SLEEP, THE BETTER YOU FUNCTION FROM SUNRISE TO SUNSET.

PLANNING FOR THE NEW DAY

I shut the light and say a prayer
Hoping that the new day will take me there
There is the place where I want to be
Where optimism is the desired outlook for me

Uplifted and strong, my journey will begin
Where I gather the will and the tools to win
A positive attitude is the shining light
Inspiration is the source for a life so bright

The sun rises and that new day is here
I welcome it with joy and good cheer
I put on my smile which I choose to wear
And dress in bright colors with great care

I go about my day using each inspirational tool
Kindness, giving, positive thinking is my rule
Mindful of myself and the emotions I feel
Making good choices and decisions so real

Obstacles may come and they'll be challenges to meet
But I can deal with them standing strong on my feet
One step at a time, staying focused and positive is the way
To have an optimistic, bright, happy and glorious day

Rita Kaufman

ROUTE 5 – WINNING WAYS TO A POSITIVELY ENERGIZED BRAIN

3 STEPS TO BOOST YOUR IMMUNE SYSTEM AND INCREASE YOUR SMILE MILEAGE

DEEP BREATHING

THE POWER OF LAUGHTER

THE POWER OF SMILES

THE COMFORT OF A HUG

MODERATE EXERCISE

PICTURE VISUALIZATION

HUMOR – THE FUNTASTIC WAY TO DEAL WITH STRESS

SMILE DOODLES TO RELIEVE EMOTIONAL STRESS AND MUSCLE TENSION

THE IDEAL WAY TO HEAL WHAT AILS YOU

LOOKING FOR HAPPINESS

Looking for happiness is what I desire
It's a goal so many aimlessly seek
Life goes fast and can be overwhelming
I want to feel strong and not to feel weak

I don't need a mansion in the suburbs
Nor do I need furs and jewels by the mile
But I do need emotional security and balance
To find joy, contentment and reasons to smile

I feel helpless when things don't go right
Though I try, I can't do enough
I work hard to grasp at solutions
But, at times, it seems really too tough

Running away from it is not an option
Closing my eyes to it is not what to do
But when I reach for my tools to guide me
It sheds light and focus on starting anew

I write things down that hurt or upset me
And then, with vigor, I tear it in strips
Leaving my hands, negativity goes with it
Along with the stress that so quickly dips

I practice deep breathing for instant relaxation
Then find a pleasant and safe place in my mind
A flower garden, beach or the waves of an ocean
A beautiful park or a sunset of the prettiest kind

These strategies and tools energize me
And give me a means to an end
Viable solutions no longer elude me
But appear with the calmness they send

Rita Kaufman

3 STEPS TO BOOST YOUR IMMUNE SYSTEM AND INCREASE YOUR SMILE MILEAGE

Step 1. Every time you wash your hands, sing or hum the tune "Happy Birthday" at least 2 times.

Step 2. Words to say while the germs go down the drain:
Today, I celebrate the first day of the rest of my life.

Step 3. Smile into the mirror for a guaranteed smile in return.

DEEP BREATHING

Rx: For defusing anger, fear, anxiety, or sadness and restoring inner biochemical balance

When you feel bored, confused, defeated, depressed, disappointed, discouraged, disgusted, downhearted, exhausted, hopeless, helpless, lonely or unloved, the cool thing to do is:

Breathe Deeply

Step 1 – Silently inhale to the count of 3

Step 2 – Hold your breath for the count of 3.

Step 3 – Say '*aaaah*' as you exhale to the count of 3.

Visualize each letter '*a*' with 2 dots and a curve.

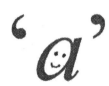

Use loosely extended fingers for counting.
Left hand fingers for inhale count.
Right hand fingers for exhale count.

Deep Breaths can be repeated as many times as it takes for your Body Systems to cool down.

The way you breathe affects the way you feel!!! Deep breathing allows your supply of smiles to grow and grow. You will feel cheerful, happy, glad, joyful, powerful, terrific, super!!!

It works, it really, really works!!! Yes, Yes, Yes!!!

THE POWER OF LAUGHTER

Laughter is the most inexpensive and most effective wonder drug.
Laughter is a universal medicine.
> Bertrand Russell

Laughter

Gives your heart and diaphragm muscles a beneficial workout.
Improves your circulation.
Fills your lungs with oxygen-rich air.
Clears your respiratory passages.
Stimulates the release of Endorphins into your bloodstream.
Reduces the tension in your Central Nervous System.

Learn to laugh at your mistakes.
Share amusing stories, and jokes that you have heard or read.

Laughter is the shortest distance between 2 People.
> Victor Borge

Laughter is free, legal, has no calories, no cholesterol, no preservatives, no artificial ingredients and is absolutely safe.
> Dale Irvin

THE POWER OF A SMILE

A smile relaxes your facial muscles and acts as a natural face-lift.
A smile produces a positively energized environment.
A smile has the power to

Send self-esteem soaring.
Make frowns disappear.
Inspire imagination.
Lead to loving relationships.
Energize one's brain and body regardless of age or gender.

Smile every time you look into the mirror!!!

A smile is a curve that sets everything straight.
> Phyllis Diller

BOTTOM LINE

**A SMILE IS THE UNIVERSAL SYMBOL FOR KINDNESS.
LET YOUR SMILE BE YOUR STYLE!!!**

A LAUGH A DAY

It's healthy to find reasons to laugh each day
And look at your life in a humorous way
Laughing perks you up and for your mind is food
To keep you happy and elevate your mood

You can laugh when you read a joke in a book
Or laugh at yourself when in the mirror you look
You can laugh when you watch a T.V. show
And laugh along with the people you know.

You can laugh at humorous cards given to you
Or laugh at monkeys doing the things that they do
You can laugh at silly steps when jumping in place
And also laugh at a friend making a funny face

Many things encourage laughing for you and for me
Embrace your laughter at the fun things you see
To ensure that your stress takes less of a toll
Try making laughter your personal goal

Rita Kaufman

THE VALUE OF SMILES

I love the many smiles I see
So therapeutic – they bring smiles to me
I happily feel my stress reducing
Looking at smiles is smile inducing

Smiles are gifts that are worth giving
They make for daily, happy living
When you willingly give smiles to those you meet
They're returned to you at home and on the street

Choose to smile with kind words to say
Along with thumbs up for a joyful day
A smile instantly changes a negative mood
And for the mind, it's a wholesome food

Smiles help the cells in our bodies thrive
And keep our focus and spirit alive
Get aboard the smile train as you embrace
A calmer, peaceful and a better place

Rita Kaufman

LEND A HAND AND A SMILE

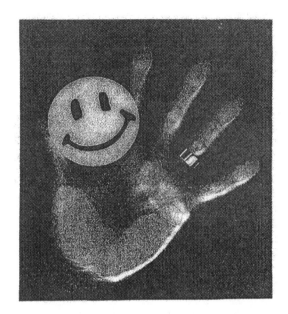

Lend a hand and a smile
To those whom you meet
You'll find life more pleasant
The more people you'll greet
Lend a hand to someone tired or in need
It will help them and also reward you indeed

It might be to help someone crossing the street
Or go to the store for food much needed to eat
It might be to fix someone's window or door
Or to peel an apple right down to its core
It might be to change a tire or hammer a nail
Or make a sandwich or get someone's mail

To lend a smile is easy and requires no skill
But when one is returned you'll find it's a thrill
A smile is a language shared by one and all
Living here or there, young or old, short or tall
It brings such joy and makes special one's day
And costs nothing at all – not even a cent to pay

Time spent together means a great deal
The warmth and good will so lovely to feel
The hand that's generously given by you
Results in shared smiles so helpful too
Thus, a hand and a smile to give and receive
During a visit and then again as you leave

Rita Kaufman

SHARE A SMILE

Share a smile with someone you meet
The feeling is great, it can't be beat
When you happily give your smile away
You'll see it come back to you each day

Give smiles to those who may be down
And maybe you'll turn their day around
Warm smiles are sincere and fit the bill
A meaningful treasure and quite a thrill

You'll feel so good and they will too
Sharing smiles are cool things to do
It's the greatest gift that you can give
It's a wonderful way for you to live

Sharing smiles can change so much
It's a beautiful way to stay in touch
Smiles are free to give, not even a dime
It can change the world - one smile at a time

Rita Kaufman

THE COMFORT OF A HUG -- A SIMPLE PAIN-FREE WORKOUT

A HUG is an important source of comfort. Aches and pains need the comfort of a hug. When you give and get a hug, you establish a reciprocal flow of positive energy. By extending your arms, you instantly release muscle tension. Give and get at least one hug each day. If no one is available, hug yourself.

MODERATE EXERCISE -- MODERATE IN FREQUENCY AND DURATION

Increases the blood and oxygen supply to your heart and lungs.
Lowers the level of carbon dioxide in your lungs.
Lowers your blood pressure.
Relieves your muscle tension.
Increases your metabolic efficiency.
Improves your learning capacity.
Improves your mood and ability to handle stressful situations.

Select an activity that you feel you will enjoy -- a 10 - 30 minute brisk walk, swimming, dancing, bicycling, yoga, tai-chi.
Seek a place that offers you fresh air, sunshine, peace, and tranquility.

DO YOU KNOW

When you sweat, you are getting rid of harmful chemicals.

PICTURE VISUALIZATION

Enjoy the Spring season all year round. Surround yourself with pictures, posters, or paintings of scenes that celebrate Spring -- the season of renewal, harmony, peace, hope, and joy.
Visualize yourself within the setting. Observe the colors. Listen to the sounds. Smell the scents.
For pleasant dreams, view the picture/ poster before going to sleep.
To have a great day, view the picture /poster upon waking.

PRETEND TO BE A KID AGAIN

You can pretend to be a kid again
And have lots of fun at play
You can look at things less seriously
And see them in a lighter way

You can jump, skip and bounce a ball
Or wiggle and jiggle around
You can play hopscotch and stickball
Or draw with chalk upon the ground

Revisiting childhood brings you smiles
As pretending can often do
Your fast-paced world will slow right down
Allowing calmness and freedom for you

Rita Kaufman

A SHORT GETAWAY

Everyone needs a little getaway
For deserved relaxation and rest
To put your hectic, busy day on hold
And, for a little while, leave the nest

Put comfy shoes and clothing on
Think positive and clear your mind
Sit on the beach, take a long walk
Or go to a park bench you may find

Your time away need not be long
An hour or so will do
Just long enough to reenergize
And make a calmer, happier you

Rita Kaufman

THE SUNSHINE WITHIN YOUR MIND

It's a cloudy, damp and rainy day
The sun has gone – it didn't stay
But there's lots of sun for you to find
Just look around within your mind

Think of something enjoyable to see
To make you smile or laugh with glee
It may be a joke or a child at play
A clown, a rainbow or a roll in the hay

It may be a photograph taken long ago
A birthday celebration that went just so
A beautiful sunset or sparkling stars in the sky
A cute little dog wagging its tail as it runs by

Whatever that special scene may be
Enjoy the moment and you will see
That in your mind the sun will shine
To make you happy and feel just fine

Rita Kaufman

HUMOR -- THE WRITE ANTIDOTE FOR ANXIETY AND DEPRESSION

THE FUNTASTIC WAY TO DEAL WITH STRESS AND INCREASE YOUR SMILE MILEAGE

When one is anxious, angry, or sad, the body generates large quantities of the hormones, adrenaline and cortisol. The power of healthy humor - smiles and laughter -- decreases the level of adrenaline and cortisol and increases the level of endorphins - the brain chemicals that make you feel good, refreshed and full of energy.

Become a Humor Reporter. Create a Humor Journal. Include:

Happy, Unique, Memorable, Outstanding Recollections, as well as laughable anecdotes, jokes, puns, riddles, quotes, double entendre headlines, funny bloopers, and newspaper ads, that you have heard or read.

Smile Starters for your Humor Journal from Laughing Matters, edited by Joel Goodman

Auto repair service ad - "Free pick-up and delivery.. Try us once and you'll never go anywhere again.

Bumper sticker - Support the right to arm bears.

A student when asked to write the numbers zero to 10, wrote: 0 - 2 - 10..

Have you ever tried the Heimlich Remover?

When you come to a fork in the road, take it. ---Yogi Berra

Many smiles a day keep the frowns away. Whenever you are having a frown day: deep breathe; reflect on a thought that makes you happy; hum a favorite tune; read, write, or say a "t" tongue twister as many times as it takes to change the frown to a smile. (excerpted from my book RHYMING RIDDLES AND TONS OF TONGUE TWISTERS FOR MILES OF SMILES)

Troy's thoughtful teacher toasted Troy's triumphant team.

Theo thinks the 33 thinkers thought thoughtful thoughts.

Ten testy testers tested ten tense teens.

Two tired teens took turns trimming the tangled tags on 33 thick towels.

Thirty trembling teenagers took ten tough tests.

Thirsty Theo tasted 30 tasty tangy tangerines. If thirsty Theo tasted 30 tasty tangy tangerines, where are the 30 tasty tangy tangerines thirsty Theo tasted?

It's time for Tim to thyme the 3 turkeys.

Ten tame, tan tigers tenderly touched 20 tiny, timid, tired turtles.

Tom was not taught to tie a taut knot.

Tucker tied 20 thick twigs with thick twine.

In your Journal, list all the things you enjoy doing. Do one fun thing for yourself each day -- write about it.

To measure your smile mileage, constantly monitor your t-bars and the level of your baseline.

BOTTOM LINE

EVERY DAY IS A NEW BEGINNING. START AND END THE DAY WITH A SMILE.
SHARE A SMILE WITH OTHERS!!! SMILES WORK WONDERS!!!

HERE'S TO YOUR GREAT DAY

Get up, get up, get out of bed
Stretch way up and nod your head

Put your smile upon your face
Wear it each day – do not erase

Give smiles to each person that you meet
It's such a nice way for you to greet

Your smile may be passed on to others
Shopkeepers, friends, sisters or brothers

It's a gift that comes right back to you
When you smile, others will too

Everyone will benefit from your smile
The pleasant feeling lasts a long while

Here's to you and to your great day
That starts and ends the share-a- smile way

Rita Kaufman

SMILE DOODLES

THE IDEAL WAY TO DEAL WITH EMOTIONAL STRESS AND MUSCLE TENSION

Doodling smiles can relieve emotional stress.
Doodling curved shapes can relieve muscle tension.

To nurture your nature and feel good from the top of your head to the tips of your toes, doodle rows and rows of e's, l's, a's and o's.
Fill the loops and circles with 2 dots and a curve.

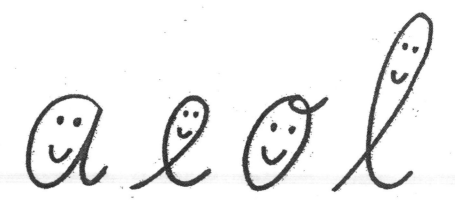

Be creative - combine the letters, connect them, separate them. The bigger the shape, the bigger the smile.

Design, display and share smile doodled messages of hope, health and happiness.

Doodle a Smiling Alphabet using the circle shaped letters – a, c, d, g, o, p, q, u.

Doodle cartoons that focus on curves and circles. Create smiling flowers and animals.

Make time for a daily dose of smile doodling.

BOTTOM LINE

A SMILE IS A CURVE THAT SETS EVERYTHING STRAIGHT.
Phyllis Diller

TWO DOTS AND A CURVE

Two dots and a curve when placed in a special way
Makes a happy face to put smiles in your day
Draw a few and then draw some more
Then look forward to the smiles that will be in store

Repeating the two dots and a curve pattern is fun
It creates relaxation and calmness for everyone
Give it a try when you're feeling tense
It's so easy to do, and there's no expense

Draw two dots and a curve – you'll be calm in a while
Draw two dots and a curve and you'll soon see a smile
Draw two dots and a curve to end anxiety and sadness
Draw two dots and a curve to feel positive gladness

Draw two dots and a curve to chase your fears away
Draw two dots and a curve and your smiles will stay
Make it a daily practice and soon you will see
Positivity will be yours and negativity will flee

Rita Kaufman

FOR INFINITE MILES OF SMILES ANY TIME OF DAY OR NIGHT

Write a series of figure "8's", in slow motion, moving from the left to the right side of the page. Turn the figure "8" on its side and you have the symbol for eternal life, serenity and harmony. Write 3 rows of the serenity symbol:

Row 1 - Place a dot and a curve in the left loop of each figure.

Row 2 - Place 2 dots and a curve in both loops of each figure.

Row 3 - Place a dot and a curve in the right loop of each figure.

You now have a smiling reminder to take the time to think, talk and write about past and present situations, events, and experiences that fill you with joy and pride as well as the sights, sounds, and scents that make you smile.

WHAT THE SMILING DOODLES HAVE TO SAY

Row 1 About The Past

Once a moment passes, it is history. One cannot change history. Energy spent dwelling on the painful past is unproductive use of time. Only past happy events are worth remembering. They have the magic power to stimulate the positive chemicals in your Brain which strengthen your Immune System.

Row 2 About The Present

The only time changes can be made is in the powerful present. Today is where the action is. Today's positive action forms the foundation for a strong future.
Each new day brings new learning experiences and endless opportunities. Spend each day seeking joy and satisfaction and there will be no room for anger and dissatisfaction. Enjoy each moment, one at a time. Focus on what is happening - not on what might happen.

Row 3 About The Future

It is impossible to predict what is ahead until you get there. If you insist on predicting, predict only positive, good things.

ADD COLOR TO YOUR SMILING DOODLES

Each person responds emotionally and physically to the sensation of color energy.

Color energy affects the chemistry of all your body systems.

Use the colors listed below when adding color to your smile doodles.

Pink Color Energy increases the blood supply to your brain and calms the nerves.

Green Color Energy lowers your blood pressure and relieves your muscle tension.

Turquoise Color Energy relieves your emotional stress and tension.

Light Blue Color Energy slows down your body metabolism and lowers your blood pressure

Purple Color Energy lowers your blood pressure and calms your nerves.

BOTTOM LINE

FOR THE TIME OF YOUR LIFE: BE IN THE PEP STATE OF MIND. KEEP ON SMILING!!!

TODAY WILL SHINE

Yesterday is history; it's all in the past
Tomorrow has yet to be seen
Today is the only day to focus on
With your actions so clear and so keen

Keep your thoughts in the present
This day alone is the one to shine
While you work, play, relax and smile
Things all around you will fall into line

Make choices with full attention and thought
And make your decisions with equal care
The result will serve you happily
With infinite fun and joy to share

Rita Kaufman

A SMILE DOODLED MESSAGE

Positively energized words and smiles make one feel calm, cool and connected.

Awareness plus humor leads to hope, health and happiness!!!

Step 1 – Write 3 rows of *aha ha-ha aaah.*
Step 2 – Take 3 deep breaths.

Step 3 - Write 3 rows of *aha ha-ha aaah.*

Step 4 - Add 2 dots and a curve to each letter "𝒶"
Step 5 – Take 3 deep breaths.
Step 6 - Repeat steps 3, 4, 5.

THE BOTTOM LINES

FEEL IT IN YOUR FINGERS
FEEL IT IN YOUR TOES
SEE HOW FAST IT REALLY, REALLY SHOWS!!!

Have fun --- Yes!!! Yes!!! Yes!!!

PEP MESSAGES TO KEEP IN MIND AND SMILE DOODLE

Love is the most powerful healing energy. Love dissolves anger, releases resentment, dispels fear and creates safety.

> Live to love and you will love to live.
> I love to laugh.
> I love to learn.
> I am living my dream.
> I live for today.
> I embrace empowering and enjoyable experiences.

Fill 'e' and 'l' loops with 2 dots and a curve. Fill a's and o's with 2 dots and a curve.

LIGHTEN UP YOUR LIFE AND FREE YOUR MIND FROM FEAR.

Smile doodle the a's, o's, e's and l's in pep words that make you smile and feel good inside and out. Use *"It Suits Me to a t" – A List of Positively Energized Words* to choose the pep words that work well for you.

FREE YOUR MIND FROM GUILT

Eliminate all 'should' and 'should have' thoughts from your mind. It places unrealistic demands on your self and results in self-directed anger, guilt and depression. Guilt is an attempt to reform the past.

Rx: TO DELETE A 'SHOULD' THOUGHT FROM YOUR MIND

Write yourself a letter giving yourself permission to forget any past painful experience. Tell yourself that it is time to stop spending energy living in the past. It is time to live in the present moment where positive change <u>can</u> take place. It is <u>OK</u> to focus on what you wish and would love to do. Now is the time to **T̲hink H̲appy T̲houghts**. (THT)

DO SMILE DOODLES

Write as many lines of the capital letters "OK" as you wish.
Add 2 dots and a curve to each letter "O".
The bigger the "O", the more space for a bigger smiles!!!

OK OK OK

BOTTOM LINE

TWO DOTS AND A CURVE GIVE YOU THE PEP TO GO WHERE YOU WISH TO GO.

FOOD FOR THOUGHT FOR AN OPTIMISTIC OUTLOOK

When you have an optimistic outlook, you feel hopeful.
When you feel hopeful, you feel

H	healthy and happy
O	optimistic and open-minded
P	patient and peaceful
E	enthusiastic and energetic
F	focused and free from fear
U	unconditional acceptance of self and others
L	love for self and others

THE WRITE, READ AND SAY WAY TO START AND END EACH DAY.

Write, read and say this statement, 3 times
   "Everything is okay in the end. If it's not okay, it is not the end."
If it is not okay, think about what positive action you can take to make it okay.

THE IDEAL WAY TO HEAL WHAT AILS YOU

Tune in to the power of musical energy. Start a collection of musical favorites.

Harmonious melodies can soothe and heal every cell in you body- your nerves, muscles, glands, heartbeat and blood pressure. Positively energized lyrics can calm your fears, lift your spirits and convert frowns and grimaces to miles of smiles and laughter.
Humming a simple childhood melody can instantly relieve emotional stress.

Your body's response to the power of musical energy can be to:
   Bend, bounce
   Clap
   Dance
   Encircle your arms
   Flex your muscles
   Glide
   Hum, hop
   Jump
   March around

Nod your head
Run, raise your arms and legs
Shake your shoulders, sing, skip, slide, snap your fingers, swing and sway,
stretch
Tap your feet, twist and turn
Whistle

My long-time favorites are:
Oh, What a Beautiful Morning
Smile
Accentuate the Positive

BOTTOM LINE

**TO FEEL GREAT, MORNING, NOON AND NIGHT, SCHEDULE DAILY
DOSES OF MUSIC.**
It works. It really, really works. Yes, yes, yes!!!

ROUTE 6 – SHARE-A-SMILE JOURNALING

SHARE-A-SMILE JOURNALING

Have fun recording and recalling joyful, humorous experiences of persons, places and events.

Share-a-Smile Memory Journaling has the magical power to:

Successfully relieve stress and serve as a never-ending source of enjoyment.

Make frowns disappear.

Inspire feelings of joy and enthusiasm.

Lead to lots of laughter.

Energize everyone's mind and body, regardless of age, gender or economic background.

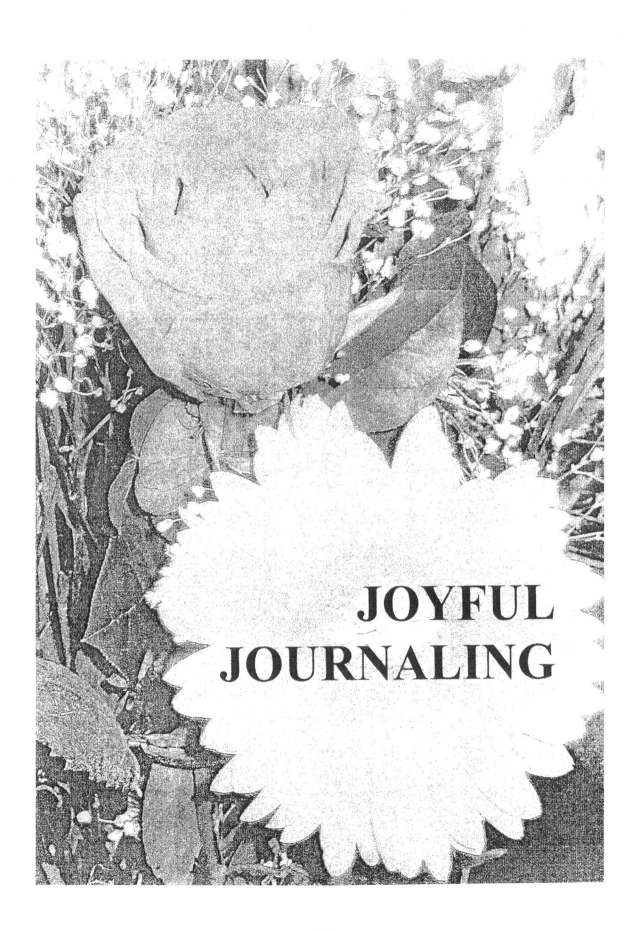

JOYFUL JOURNALING

To the Reader

Who hasn't, at some time, felt overwhelmed, bored, anxious, fearful, or worried?

With the complexities of daily living, the state of today's world and our own individual concerns, a positive approach to life is beneficial, healing and open to joyous possibilities.

The poems sprinkled within the pages of the Routes are intended to provide inspiration, choices and possible solutions to challenges while navigating through life's ups and downs. The focus is on an energizing, empowering and positive outlook, resulting in satisfaction, laughter happiness and peace of mind.

The poems in the Joyful Journaling section are intended to bring to the forefront the observation and awareness of pleasurable moments. Thinking, writing and reminiscing about these joyful moments stimulates the body and brain, enriches quality of life, reduces stress and makes a healthier and happier you!

The poems were originally conceived as a way of finding new dimension, personal well-being and optimism in my life. It is my hope that sharing the expressed thoughts and feelings lighten your own heart and make it sing with joy.

Rita Kaufman

With pen in hand, I choose to write
Of many things that bring delight,
Of things that are stress free,
Things that bring joy to me.
          Rita Kaufman

OUR SPECIAL BOND

Photography is a form of creativity
A means of expression from within
It's more than just capturing
memories
But opens up a world and lets you in

My dad loved photography
It was his passion from the start
His many skills rubbed off on me
I treasure this bond within my heart

Just like my dad, my camera's close
From its lens I look and see
The colors, shapes and forms of life
Of the world that surrounds me

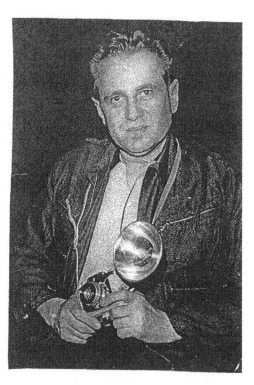

I see true meaning in the eyes
Of people, friends and family
I try to capture all of this
And with respect treat all I see

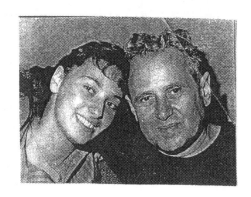

Like my dad, I generously give
This gift that's meant to share
Photos of memories to embrace
Tokens of how much I really care

Their smiles make me feel good inside
The rewards so meaningful and strong
The gift my dad passed on to me
Became part of the world in which I belong

I see his face in front of me
His camera held with delight
I thank him for this legacy
That makes my life so bright.

Rita Kaufman

(Past memories of a loved one are comforting thoughts to warm the heart.)

RECAPTURED MEMORIES

It's especially nice to go down memory lane
To revisit memories and recapture the same
To rekindle the joys safely stored in your mind
Back to those days and the memories you'll find

Memories of college and friends once held dear
Memories of past jobs in your chosen career
Memories of people whose paths you've crossed
Memories of all those connections you've lost

Find an old address book and pick up the phone
Even if it's an action taken by you all alone
The effort and journey may be worthwhile
One that may ultimately bring you a smile

Rita Kaufman

HAPPY MEMORIES

Recall your happy memories of childhood past
Where in your mind and heart they'll always last
The ones that make you smile or shed a happy tear
Those of friendship and family that remain so clear

Licking pudding from the bowl prepared by your mom
Playing hopscotch and tag with friends that come
Hugging your parents as you leave for the school
Smiles from your teacher because you follow her rule

Successful school years, summers and more
Malteds and ice cream from the corner store
Graduations, diplomas and the feeling of pride
Your beautiful wedding as a groom or a bride

The first cry heard from your daughter or son
Accolades from projects that were so well done
Happily think of these memories now and then
Smile and enjoy the feeling over and over again

Rita Kaufman

CHILDHOOD SUMMER DAYS

I think of summer days and childhood gone by so fast
Remembering the fun we had, hoping it would always last

Report cards were given, the bell rang and school was out
"It's summer vacation", we would all enthusiastically shout

Some friends went to camp, and to the bus they'd eagerly run
While others, like myself, were happy to enjoy the Brooklyn sun

The days were hot and the nights were cool
Play, fun and relaxation was the followed rule

My mom and grandmother sat with neighbors to chat
I worked on my horse rein, lanyard and things like that

When the ice cream truck came by, ringing its bell
My favorite flavor, in a cup, I would happily tell

Finishing the ice cream, I quickly rinsed the lid
And looked for the picture on it, when I was a kid

I took my pencil and pad and sat down to draw
The cartoon on the lid, hopefully, without a flaw

I went to the beach with friends and had lots of fun
And watched television at night with everyone

I played hit the penny, stick ball and had many a race
Board games with friends put a smile on my face

Monopoly and Clue were the two I liked best
We'd play for hours without taking a rest

When summer days were gone; I looked forward to Fall
But not without pleasant memories for me to recall

They're stored safely in the bank within my mind
And know that right inside, these memories I can find

Cherished memories bring joy in just a little while
Whenever we may need a lift or an extra, special smile

Rita Kaufman

BIRTHDAYS

The pleasure of a birthday is one to behold
Whether we're five or ten or a hundred years old
Many thoughts emerge as each birthday we see
Then make a wish and blow out the candles with glee

The very young wish for all kinds of toys
Teens wish for dates with special girls or boys
Young adults wish for cars and jobs that fit them just so
Older folks wish for good health and that happiness glow

Cards are sent with love and admiration
Phone calls are made all over the nation
Parties are planned with decorations galore
Icing on cakes, presents, well-wishes and more

But birthdays come and then they go
With good times enjoyed by those who know
That a birthday is just a number, not a yardstick used for
measure
But instead a very special day to rejoice in and treasure

Rita Kaufman

GRANDCHILDREN

The strain of life is minimized
When my grandchildren smile at me
The aches and pains no longer hurt
When they climb upon my knee

We enjoy each other's company
And lovingly share our day
We smile and laugh so happily
As we join together in play

I feel that I can meet challenges
When I hear them laugh with glee
I feel alive and energized
When they are close to me

Rita Kaufman

A PRE-KINDERGARTEN SHOW

We eagerly await the show to start
The audience is ready to do their part
Onto the stage the young stars walk
Everyone is quiet and no one will talk
We see their waves and smiling faces
They watch us sitting as they take their places

We look at each child and our own girl or boy
And before long, we happily shed tears of joy
The children are young – just four years old
But they sing and dance as they've been told
They entertain us in such a wonderful way
And give us all a joyous and memorable day

They're very cute and perform so great
To hug and kiss them, we can't wait
We're proud and smile from ear to ear
This culmination of a special year
Now on they move to the next grade
We're grateful for the growth they've made

Rita Kaufman

(This was written after watching our grandson perform in his Pre-K Graduation show)

A CHILD'S PICTURE

Our grandson drew a picture of himself today
His bright eyes and glowing smile had so much to say
It was a picture of wonder, joy and happiness galore
Of excitement, energy and confidence to soar

He's young, his world is safe and he's okay
We pray that it will continue to stay that way
Society is filled with fear, negativity and distress
How do we protect our children from this unrest

We must believe and keep the light within us well lit
Be aware, proactive, on target and emotionally fit
So our challenges can be met with enthusiasm and hope
With positive energy, love and strength to successfully cope

Rita Kaufman

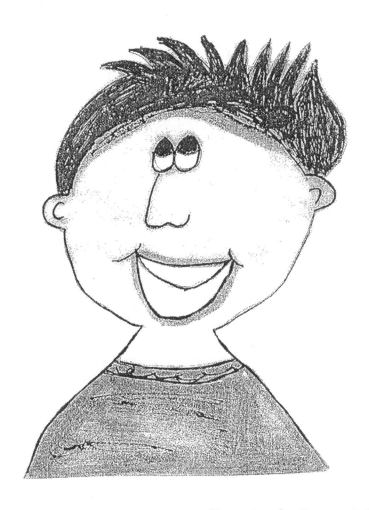

Drawing by Bryan Acker – Age 6

RUSTY AND ME

I sat on the sofa watching T.V.
With tired eyes drifting away
My cat sat down next to me
So comfy and planning to stay

Back and forth, I stroked his fur gently
It was so silky and soft to the touch
He closed his eyes as he purred softly
As if to say, "thank you so much"

This comforting gift was mutual
He calmed me as I did him
Together we were in dreamland
Background T.V. and the light so dim

He woke up and looked toward me
Took a long stretch with ease and grace
Then turned to gently lick my hand
As I smiled at his adorable face

He gracefully jumped off the sofa
Our time together was done
For me the memory lingered
Of Rusty and me – together as one

Rita Kaufman

(Precious time spent relaxing with a family pet can gently soothe the soul.)

MY CAT BRINGS ME JOY

I smiled with joy the other day
Watching my little cat at play
He was having so much fun
But he was not the only one

He swatted a bug upon the wall
Then chased yarn throughout the hall
He climbed into a paper sack
And rolled around on his back

He played with a feather on the kitchen floor
And with the mail that came through the door
I smiled and laughed at his curiosity
It was such a wonderful sight to see

He came over to me for a tasty treat
A bonus for a day that was upbeat
He gently sat upon my lap
And prepared himself for a nap

His soft purring felt very good
He was so easily understood
And though he was unable say
I knew he had a real nice day

Rita Kaufman

MY CUTE LITTLE CAT

My cute, little cat likes to play
With a ping pong ball all day
He kicks the ball with his paw
Then chases it around some more

Looking for food, he wants to eat
His yummy salmon or chicken treat
Then he climbs upon my lap
And cuddles into a nice, long nap

I love to hear his gentle purr
And slowly pet his soft, soft fur
He wakes up with a stretch or two
And thinks about what he should do

I get his ping pong ball and say
"Come over here – come on let's play"
When done, he plops upon the rug
And waits for me to give a hug

He's so adorable, anyone can see
Especially when he "kisses" me
He adds happiness to each day
In his own unique and special way

Rita Kaufman

THE FLOOR ATE AND THE CAT PLAYED

The cleaning service left and the house was so clean
Everything shined and was in place like a dream
I walked into the kitchen for a blueberry snack
My plate was ready and I took a spoon from the rack

The freezer door opened and blueberries fell to the floor
They went flying all over, even way down to the door
The frozen berries bounced, going in every direction
Dining room, hallway, and in the kitchen, each section

Our little cat thought that chasing them was a game
I ran to pick up each berry while calling his name
Then to distract him, I opened salmon on the counter top
But suddenly it fell to the floor and I heard a big "plop"

Oh, no – once again he's here, our playful, curious cat
And licked up the salmon from the floor and the mat
Frazzled and stressed, I took a bowl for cereal to eat
Nothing very special – but at that moment, a treat

I reached in the shelf, but the cereal box slipped
Flakes all over the floor and I almost tripped
In came our cat, thinking more games to play
He was so excited about his adventurous day

The once clean floor ate such a variety of food
To wash it now, I was so not in the mood
But I took out the sweeper, the water and mop
And again the house was clean from bottom to top

Rita Kaufman

POEMS TO WELCOME A PET SITTER

The following poems were written for our cat sitter, Stacey.
Upon entering our home, Stacey, would find a poem "written" by Rusty, our
cat. She would tell us that they always bring smiles to her face. Welcoming her
in this manner makes me feel good as well – it's nice to provide a reason for
someone to smile!!!

Dear Stacey,

My folks are packed and going on vacation
And Stacey, you and I can have a celebration
I'll watch you wrap your holiday gifts with glee
Then before you go, please leave a treat for me

I'll wait for you to visit me each day
And when I see you I'll meow "hooray"
Thanks for taking such good care of me
You're the best sitter there could ever be

> Love,
> Rusty

Dear Stacey,

Everything's in place – my bed, litter and many a treat
Thanks for your visits – your personality can't be beat
Please keep my water fresh and give me treats galore
Then I'll purr and be your furry friend forever more

> Love,
> Rusty

Dear Stacey,

My folks left great snacks for you
Cookies, chips and healthy fruit too
The refrigerator is the place to be
There are yummy things to see

I look around and enjoy the view
My favorite is salmon and turkey too
I like to eat them in treats as well
Give me some and I'll feel just swell

You're my friend and I love you so
I like when you pet me – I'm sure you know
I'll stay close to you and purr a song
And await your next visit – please don't be long

                    Love,
                    Rusty

Dear Stacey,

Two, four, six, eight, ten
You'll soon be here again
I have my ping pong ball today
I hope that you would like to play
You have such a happy smile
I love when you stay here a while
The door will open – hip, hip hooray
And then my day will be A-okay

                    Love,
                    Rusty

Dear Stacey,

When you're here to take care of me
I happily meow and purr with glee
Give me treats for an added touch
Your furry friend likes them so much
I welcome your visits every day
Please relax with me, if that's okay

Love,
Rusty

Dear Stacey,

I'm glad that you are here today
Here's my feather, if you'd like to play
I hope that you'll give me a treat
One that's yummy and crunchy to eat
When you leave and go home for the night
I'll go to sleep as you shut off the light
Then wait for tomorrow, as I always do
To greet you, meow and gently purr too

Love,
Rusty

Dear Stacey,

Sitting on the couch is where I like to be
It makes me happy when you sit with me
I may fall asleep on you, but don't feel bad
When you treat me so nicely - I feel so glad

Love,
Rusty

TARKY

Tarky, our pet Golden is part of our family
He's so cute, lovable and as loyal as can be
He's our family's cuddly and furry little boy
And gives unconditional love and such joy

He sits by the door and gets excited seeing our car
We watch as he wags his tail and thrills us by far
Our grandchildren open the door as he runs to greet us
We eagerly hug him and with a smile make a fuss

We go into the house to visit and talk
But Tarky patiently awaits Papa's walk
He goes for his leash and meets Papa's eyes
Then they walk together with love and close ties

Later I sit on the couch with Tarky so near
Petting and rubbing his belly which he loves so dear
We remember him as a puppy, but now he has grown
But still likes to be near us as he chews his yummy bone

He looks into our eyes which say so much
It pulls at our heartstrings with the warmest of touch
He's Tarky, our Golden who's affectionate and sweet
Just being with him gives each day a very special treat

Rita Kaufman

These photographs are examples of calming, enjoyable scenes that are ideal for relaxation and reduction of stress. They are the places where some of my poems gained inspiration and were written.

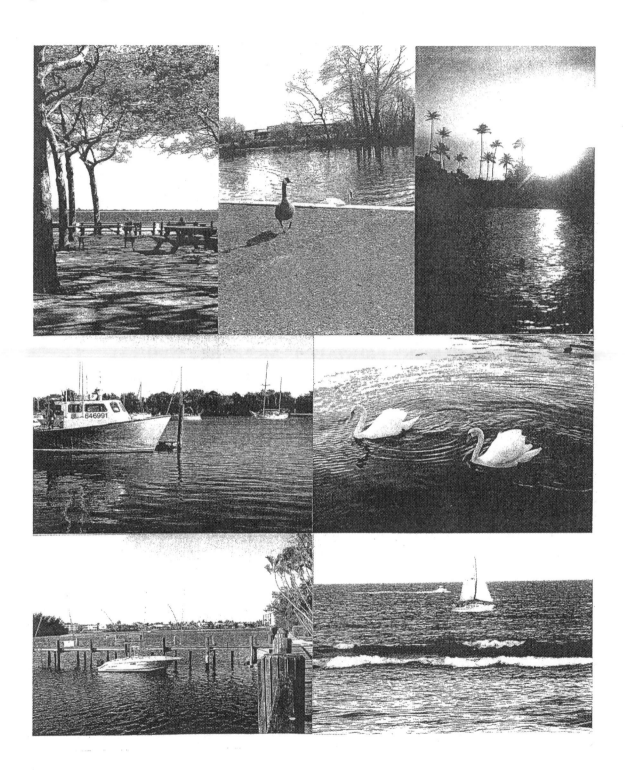

RELAXING BY THE INTRACOASTAL

The Intracoastal – a beautiful place to be seen
With the water so blue and the grass so green
The air so clear and the leaves so still
For relaxation and peace, it fits the bill

Boats gently glide, each upon a delicate wave
Presenting a glorious boat parade
Enthusiasts sail or water ski
Clearly the place they want to be

For me, my body is relaxed and so is my mind
Enriching calmness of the very best kind
Now I'm ready to resume the rest of my day
So fully recharged in a most positive way

Rita Kaufman

A QUIET DAY AT THE BEACH

The sun began to shine on this Monday in May
So beautiful after morning rain started the day
The beach is empty – only a few folks are here
Just two children playing – one far and one near

The weekend crowds have all gone home
No one to sit and no one to roam
The ocean waves flow gently as they go
Forming a pattern, some high and some low

A lone bird perched on wood in the sand
While some birds fly and others land
Watching the view and the vision I see
A quiet beach day, so peaceful to me

Rita Kaufman

OUR CARRIBEAN VACATION

The Caribbean palm trees enhance the beauty of these days
While enjoying each detail in oh, so many ways
The green color, the sway in the wind and the glow from the sun
Along with the beach, pool and music - we delight in each one

Our beautiful room with its sunny balcony to see
Inspires peace, relaxation and harmony in me
Delightful restaurants, each with a delectable cuisine
Delivers exactly in the way you hope it would seem

Friends surround us and share in good cheer
Adding to the wonder of this vacation, so clear
Guests and staff welcome and greet each other with a smile
Thus sprinkling the day ahead with happiness all the while

But now it's time to return to New York and head for the plane
With mounds upon mounds of snow, ice and even some rain
The pool, palm trees and beach is etched forever in my mind
To call upon, dream about, while reachable and so easy to find.

Rita Kaufman

OUR HOTEL STAY

We're here to check-in and take our key
Then look around for things to see
A staff member greets us with a smile
And says, "Glad you're here with us a while"

We sit at the breakfast buffet after leaving our suites
And look forward to the array of delicious treats
The skillful omelet chef is ready and awaits his line
Ham, mushrooms, onion, tomato, cheese – he looks for your sign

Young children pull the lever and Froot Loops fill their bowl
Some may add a banana, a half or a whole
They love the colors and Cheerios too
But retrieving them is the game, and fun to do

Yogurt and fruit, along with prunes for those in need
Sausage, bacon, potatoes, eggs - all yummy indeed
Bagels, English muffins and bread galore
Muffins, donuts, pancakes and much more

Smiles on our faces and full bellies too
It's time for sun, enjoying nothing to do
Off to the exercise room which is inviting
Feeling good while burning calories is exciting

The grounds are beautiful and the pool is as well
It's fun to swim and relax in the hot tub for a spell
Each day here is spent happily in much the same way
We thank the gracious hotel staff for our enjoyable stay

Rita Kaufman

THOUGHTS IN THE NIGHT

It's time for bed
I fall asleep fine
It doesn't take long
Hardly any time

I just watch the clock
My sleep won't stay
Now what shall I do
Too soon for a new day

So with paper and pen
I write words and rhymes
Of thoughts and people
And of special times

I close my tired eyes
Trying to ease my mind
Thinking of pleasant dreams
And ultimately I find

Morning sleep does come
It's the very best kind
A new poem is complete
That last night left behind

Rita Kaufman

DESIRES

Desires run the gamut from small to large
Material and emotional thoughts take charge

Some material desires are needed for balance and dreams
But those that enrich your heart are more valued it seems

One may desire a fur coat, vacation or car
For me, peace and harmony outweigh these by far

Some may desire rich and high caloric food all week
Energy-boosting, healthy choices is what I seek

Others may desire jewelry, expensive clothing or art
Peace within my family is what I'd put in my cart

Still others desire titles, prestige and social acclaim
For me, having self-confidence and esteem is my aim

Being calm, happy, content and worry-free
Productive and well-liked are desires for me

Rita Kaufman

ROUTE 7 – PEP THOUGHTS TO KEEP IN MIND

CHOICES

CHOOSE TO HAVE POSITIVE HABITS

WHY ONE IS SIGNIFICANT

ONE MORE TRY CAN DO IT

SOME THOUGHTS ABOUT THE WORDS – TO-TOO-TWO

ZERO IN ON THE POSITIVE SIDE OF MISTAKES

THE IDEAL WAY TO SOLVE YOUR PROBLEMS

THE IDEAL WAY TO ESTABLISH SATISFYING RELATIONSHIPS

FOOD FOR THOUGHT ABOUT THE WORD "LIKE"

EXPANDING ON THE MEANING OF LOL

TIMELY FACTS

MNEMONICALLY SPEAKING

PEP ONE-LINERS THAT CAN POSITIVELY REPLACE TNT

RX FOR PEP, HOPE, HEALTH AND HAPPINESS

A DAILY 25 MINUTE, 5 STEP BEDTIME ROUTINE FOR GETTING A GOOD NIGHT'S SLEEP

MOTIVAIONAL TEXT MESSAGES

CHOICES – CHOICES -- AND MORE CHOICES

From the minute you get up to the minute you go to sleep, you are constantly making choices.

Do I choose to wake up early or late?

What color and kind of clothes do I choose to wear?

Do I choose to have long or short hair?

Do I choose to read?

What books, magazines, papers do I choose to read?

What t.v. shows do I choose to watch?

What games do I choose to play?

What kind of music do I choose to listen to?

What kind of friends do I choose to have?

Whom do I choose to talk to when I have a problem?

How do I choose to feel and act when I make a mistake?

How do I choose to handle my feelings when I am angry, frustrated or worried?

What do I choose to eat and drink for breakfast, lunch, dinner, and snack time?

You are responsible for all the choices you make in your lifetime. You always have choices. Every choice affects your body chemistry. Your choices determine how well you will function.

BOTTOM LINE

GOOD CHOICES MAKE FOR A POSITIVE ATTITUDE.

CHOOSE TO HAVE POSITIVE HABITS

When you repeatedly practice doing something in a certain way, you form a habit. The more you reinforce, or use the habit, the stronger it becomes. Positively charged habits allow your body systems to function with maximum efficiency. Negatively charged habits destroy the chemical balance of your body systems. No one is born with habits. All habits are learned. It takes time to form a habit. The length of time to learn a new habit varies for each person. For some, it may be a month. For some, it may be several months.

C P R FORMULA FOR POSITIVE HABIT PROGRAMMING
Commitment + Consistency + Patience + Practice + Repetition + Reinforcement

BOTTOM LINE
CHOOSE TO BE THE BEST YOU CAN BE!!!

EVERYDAY CHOICES

You can look at each day being positive or not
But, without fail, the positive is the best choice you've got

Situations have choices of at least two or more
Evaluate each possibility and the path that's in store

You can choose foods that are both greasy and fried
And then contend with the feeling of guilt that's inside

Or on the same empty plate you can choose to take
Salad, fish, veggies or the healthy chicken you make

You can stay in bed and let the day go by
Or dress up brightly and give a smile a try

You can listen to the negative side of your inner voice
Or let the uplifting sound of music be your choice

You can let the hustle and bustle of life sound its alarm
Or choose to close your eyes and feel the calm

You can dwell on things that bring forth anxiety and fear
Or choose to be surrounded by thoughts of good cheer

So ponder your choices because they're yours to make
But remember your feelings and moods are at stake

Then believe in these choices and from them don't stray
And the result will be a much happier you all the way

Rita Kaufman

ONGOING CHALLENGES

If you face a minor ongoing challenge
Like hard to control eating or portion size
Gambling, drinking or over your head shopping
There are things you may choose to realize

Put all things in proper perspective
Beating yourself up surely won't do
Make a list of alternate choices
And use them each day to get through

Place affirmations around to assist you
Ask family and friends for their support too
Find varied fun activities to amuse you
And appropriate solutions that also may do

There still may be times that you fall
Then pick yourself up and happily view
Your goals, strengths and determination
And joyfully begin starting anew

Rita Kaufman

WHY ONE IS SIGNIFICANT

There is only one One.

One is always first.

There is only One of you. No other One has your unique combination of physical and personality traits, characteristics, abilities, and talents.

No One can ever take another One's place.

Each One counts.

Each One has a significant role to play in life.

Each One is a teacher.

Each One influences someone.

Each One sets an example.

Each One is a role model.

It takes one step to effect change.

You can successfully deal with life if you take one day at a time, and focus on one issue or task at a time.

You have won when you believe you are a significant One!!!

It takes only One to make a difference.

BOTTOM LINE

BE THE ONE WHO CAN MAKE A DIFFERENCE!!!

ONE MORE TRY CAN DO IT!!!

When you think that you have had it, and are ready to give up and pack it in
    Try one more time.

When you are sure that you will never succeed
    Try one more time.

When you think it is impossible, too hard to do, and it will never work
    Try one more time.

When you think that it will never happen
    Try one more time.

When you think that all is lost and it will never get better
    Try one more time.

When you think that you have reached the end of your rope and there is no place to turn
    Try one more time.

When you think that you will never win
    Try one more time.

If you don't try one more time, you will never know if you might have won!!!

SOME THOUGHTS ABOUT THE WORDS - to, too, two

Small words -- same sound -- big difference in meaning!!!

"To" is a preposition meaning forward in the direction of. "To" gets you to where you want to go.

"Too" is an adverb meaning excessively. "Too" tells you that an extreme is present. Too much or too little of anything is not good. Too soon or too late is poor timing.

"Too" has two "o's". Because too has one "o" too many, it prevents you from getting to where you want to go.

"Two" is a noun or adjective meaning more than one and less than three.

If "one" is enough, do you think "two" is one too many and the beginning of too much?

ZERO IN ON THE POSITIVE SIDE OF MISTAKES

All Human Beings make mistakes. It is okay to make mistakes. A mistake is a signal that there is an existing deficiency or weakness. There is a need to remedy the existing deficiency.

Mistakes are opportunities for learning to take positive action to prevent a recurrence.

BOTTOM LINE

THE MISTAKE HAS SERVED AS A STEPPING-STONE TO LEARNING, GROWING AND ACHIEVING.

THE IDEAL WAY TO SOLVE YOUR PROBLEMS

Problems are here to stay. They are a part of Life. Problems are as unique as Individuals.

What is a problem for one, may not be a problem for another.

You have a problem when you experience feelings of anxiety, fear, frustration, anger, sadness, or guilt.

You are the only one who really knows when you have a problem. You are the only one who really knows how you feel. You are the only one who can identify, define and solve your problem.

The shortest distance between identifying problems and reaching realistic solutions is keeping your eyes focused on specific facts, issues, circumstances, and actions.

Specific questions that can help you to identify, define your problem issues and yield solutions are: "what" and "when".

What is my problem? What realistic positive action am I willing to take to solve my problem?

When is the appropriate time to begin my Positive Action Plan?

When is the appropriate time to evaluate the success of my Positive Action Plan?

Every solution is always subject to change, revision, and improvement. Life is in a constant state of flux. Nothing ever stays the same. Problems are challenges -- opportunities for change, growth, and discovery.

BOTTOM LINE

EACH PROBLEM SOLVED IS A VICTORY!!!

IMPORTANT NOTE!!!

Do not make a POSITIVE ACTION PLAN when you are feeling angry, anxious, or frustrated. Negative feelings cause a chemical imbalance in your Body Systems, and interfere with your ability to plan positive action. Take time out to restore your chemical balance. Take slow deep breaths to calm down and relax.

THE IDEAL WAY TO ESTABLISH SATISFYING RELATIONSHIPS

An individual can only speak from his /her own viewpoint, which is based upon his/her own unique experiences, ideas, beliefs and feelings. Your feelings, words, and actions must match. Say what you really feel and mean. Mean what you say. Do what you say you mean.

Focus on accuracy. Seek answers to "who", "what", "when", "where", "how".

Focus on one specific at a time -- a specific behavior, condition, event, feeling, issue, need, problem, situation, or individual.

Beware of words that fail to be specific or accurate -- generalizations, speculations, rumors, gossip, hearsay.

Each individual is entitled to express his/her own opinions.

"I" messages express your viewpoint and do not lead to confrontations.

Sentence starters for accurate stress-free communication:

In my opinion, _____

From my point of view, _____

I believe _____

I feel _____

I think _____

Beware of messages that begin with the word "You". "You" messages point an accusing finger and generate feelings of resistance and hostility.

Every individual needs his/her feelings to be acknowledged, accepted, heard, understood, and validated.

Be a PAL -- a Patient, Accurate Listener.

By accepting the fact that each individual is entitled to his/her own unique viewpoint, you are allowing the Speaker to verbally express his/her angry, sad, anxious feelings in a safe non-threatening environment. Maintain eye contact. Focus on the words that reflect the Speaker's inner feelings. Words are subject to individual interpretation. To avoid misinterpretation, it is important for the Listener to clarify and confirm his/her understanding as to the accuracy of the message heard.

Sentence starter for accurate clarification:

It seems to me that you are feeling _____

because _____..

The Speaker can agree or disagree. If the Speaker disagrees, further clarification is needed.

After the Speaker has finished expressing his/her feelings, offer support and encouragement. Ask, "What can I do to help?"

IMPORTANT TO NOTE:

The role of a Patient Accurate Listener (PAL) is not to advise, agree, analyze, approve, comment, correct, criticize, discredit, evaluate, interrupt, judge, or tease.

MARRIAGE

A marriage is a partnership between two
Each helping the other in all that they do
To make each happy and also fulfilled
To share the values that both have instilled

Though there are two, it becomes a union of one
Together at night and in the daylight sun
The aim is to please and bring each other smiles
Whether at home or travelling across many miles

A thread of togetherness woven solid and tight
Creating a tapestry so precious and right
A marriage based on love and respect is ideal
Only then can the marriage wear the quality seal

Rita Kaufman

JUST QUIETLY LISTEN

As much as you'd like to
As much as you try
You can't change someone
On that you can rely

You're always well-meaning
And love them more than life
But trying to change them
Brings tension and strife

Living each day is not easy
Looking for peace and for joy
But living the life of others
Makes it harder for <u>you</u> to enjoy

Patiently and quietly listen
Stay close and stay near
Advise only when wanted
With your support very clear

Step back and relax
Deep breathe for a while
Embrace life as it goes on
Each day with a smile

Rita Kaufman

FINDING PEACE IN YOUR LIFE

What is the way to find peace in your life
When you feel the pain of others cut like a knife
When it's difficult to help people you love so dear
With their frustration, sadness, anguish or fear

It's a feeling so helpless – a feeling so blue
How can we handle it – what can we do
We can validate their feelings and lend a kind ear
And hold our advice until asked with words so clear

We can think positive thoughts from the start
And control only these as we do our part
We can take deep breaths and gently say
I wish you well and am here for you today

We can be supportive and seek words so right
Embrace and comfort them with all our might
We can hope that their future life will reign supreme
And look forward to tomorrow with a smile and a dream

Rita Kaufman

FAMILY

The closeness of family is important
And should be priority number one
Treat all with respect, love and devotion
All through from morning until day is done

A phone call, email or sent photo
A line or two dropped in the mail
A kind word, hug or "I love you"
That's what family life should entail

Enjoy a school play or graduation
A birthday or holiday to share
A vacation taken together
All show your concern and your care

Take pride in each other's accomplishments
Feel joy from each other's success
Lend a shoulder to lean on when needed
And help to clean up each other's mess

Everyone has a daily agenda
Everyone has a life to live
But never lose sight of your family
And always be available to give

Enjoy cherished memories collected
Stories and letters of old
Photos and home movies taken
And treasured thoughts of wisdom retold

So look toward each family member
And leave their faults far behind
Let each interaction be special
And value the qualities you'll find

Being part of a family is heartwarming
And worth all the effort you spend
Enjoy the spirit, fun and the laughter
Each time you see them, from beginning to end

Rita Kaufman

A LETTER TO A FRIEND

Choose to write a letter to a friend
It's worthwhile time for you to spend
Tell her that you really care
With words so kind that you share

Think of a memorable past event
Or a fun occasion together spent
Tell her what she means to you
Maybe plan something nice to do

Tell her how you spend your day
What interests you in a special way
Keep her up to date with your family
Invite her to send photos for you to see

Keep your friendship warm and strong
It's good to know that you belong
A solid friendship is so dear
She may know, but it's nice to hear

Rita Kaufman

THE GIFT OF GIVING

There's a reachable goal and a wonderful way to live
That's attained when you lend a hand or generously give
It's so easy to do and it doesn't cost a cent
But your efforts are appreciated and your time is well spent

You can give a pat on the back and a compliment or two
A caring hand-written note or a phone call from you
You can share acts of kindness and words that bring joy
Or your own special skill that others can employ

You can make the day of a salesperson or bus driver on your way
By the smile on your face or the words that you say
Giving need not be large in scale - small doses will do
Ideas are many and plentiful and are clearly in view

Age makes no difference – whether a person is young or old
Smiles occur when something kind is done or something nice is told
You just have to be ready, motivated and willing to give
And then rewards will be yours when in this way you live

Rita Kaufman

IN PURSUIT OF PEACE

Is peace for our world an impossible dream
It seems to be replaced with hatred and war
Where is the harmony and living as one
And our environment clean to its core

Men before us have had this dream
Hopefully, our children will have it too
With peaceful thoughts and kind words for all
And positive interactions being the ones to do

To begin, find a place of peace within yourself
With feelings of trust, love, satisfaction and hope
To enable you to treat family, friends and beyond
With kindness, respect and a helping hand to cope

Accomplishing this is not an easy task
But, with desire, we have the power for sure
Person to person – country to country
A viable new world will emerge and soar

Rita Kaufman

FOOD FOR THOUGHT ABOUT THE WORD "LIKE"

When used as a preposition, "like" means "similar", "being the same as" and is used for making comparisons.

YOU are Unique. You are not like anybody else.

It is not possible to compare anyone or anything that is unique.

When used as a verb, "like" means "to enjoy", "to be fond of".

THE WAY TO GET YOUR HEAD TO GET AHEAD

Create a Smile File.

List your unique personality traits, abilities and talents. Refer to the list to complete the 3rd line of the following verse:

> I like what I see
>
> When I look at me.
>
> I like and appreciate _____.

Every time you look into the mirror, recite the 3-line verse.

Add a smile and end with Yes!!! Yes!!! Yes!!!

List all the activities that you like to do. Refer to your list to schedule a daily dose of a likeable activity. Recall and record your enjoyed activity before going to sleep.

BOTTOM LINE

BE AWARE OF WHAT IT IS THAT YOU SAY TO YOURSELF.
THE MORE YOU WRITE, THE BETTER YOU FEEL AND THE BETTER YOU SLEEP!!!

EXPANDING ON THE MEANING OF THE NEW WORD IN THE DICTIONARY

LOL
Lots Of Love
Lots Of Laughter
Lots Of Learning
Lots Of Listening

1. Select an LOL message to write and recite.
2. Write three lines of the LOL text message. Punctuate the message with an exclamation point!!!

3. Recite the message three times.
For increased vim, vigor and vitality, add the words yes!!! yes!!! yes!!!

What differences do you see in lines 1, 2, and 3 of the written text?
How does you voice sound after reciting your LOL text message?
Are you now ready to really laugh out loud?

BOTTOM LINE
MAKE TIME FOR A DAILY DOSE OF LOL MESSAGES

TIMELY FACTS

Each individual has his/her own unique inner biological clock – a sense of timing, and body rhythm. Your sense of timing depends on your unique basic personality temperament. Your glands produce hormones and chemicals that control your unique inner 24-hour biological clock, and determine how many hours your body needs for sleeping, waking and eating.

Sufficient rest is essential to balance your inner body rhythm. To relieve stress, schedule reasonable and realistic periods of time to eat, work, sleep, relax and exercise.

If you spend too much time thinking about past painful issues, you are governed by feelings of anger. If you spend too much time thinking about events that will happen in the future, you are governed by fear.

Productive use of your time, produces a feeling of competency.

Respect the importance of Time. Each moment is an opportunity that is never repeated. It takes one moment to initiate a change that can affect the direction of your whole Life. It takes one shared moment to change relationships. It takes one moment to provide the Hope for a good tomorrow.

Successful outcomes are based upon good choices and good timing. Good timing requires realistic planning. Time, patience, and practice make everything better. Your timing is off when you begin too soon, too late, or spend too much time in one area of activity.

As long as there is life, there is time to:

appreciate who you are and what you have, believe in yourself, change, defuse your level of stress and tension, enjoy life, free yourself from the painful feelings of anger, sadness and fear, grow, get in touch with what you see, hear, smell and taste, help yourself, initiate positive action, learn new skills, laugh, monitor what is required for maintaining balance and moderation, nurture your needs, open your mind to available options, positively energize for optimum functioning, quell the inner qualms, reorganize, simplify your life, treasure each moment, understand yourself, value yourself, win, express your feelings, zero in on the specifics that can satisfy your unique needs.

PEP MESSAGES TO KEEP IN MIND

MNEMONICALLY SPEAKING - A DEVICE FOR REMEMBERING MEANINGFUL CONCEPTS WITHIN A WORD

PEP lives and thrives within a Satisfying <u>Relationship</u>

R	Respect, Responsibility
E	Enthusiasm
L	Love
A	Acceptance of what is
T	Trust
I	Insight
O	Open-mindedness
N	Nurturing nature
S	Safety, Stability, Smiles
H	Healthy Sense of Humor
I	Integrity
P	Patience, Positive Attitude

WHAT IS TO BE FOUND IN A GOOD <u>LIFE</u>

L	Learning, Listening, Loving, Laughing
I	Ideas, Independence, Integrity, Insight
F	Freedom From Fear And Frustration
E	Enjoyable Experiences

ISSUES IMPORTANT TO <u>FOCUS</u> IN ON

F	Feelings, Facts
O	Options, Order, Organization
C	Consistent Constructive Change
U	Understanding
S	Specifics

A <u>SMILE</u> HAS THE POWER TO

Send self-esteem soaring.

Make frowns disappear.

Inspire feelings of hope, joy, and inner peace.

Lead to lots of love and laughter.

Energize the brain and body regardless of one's age, gender, or economic background.

GET HIGH ON HOPE.

Health and Happiness

Optimism

Patience and Perseverance

Enthusiasm

PEP ONE-LINERS THAT CAN POSITIVELY REPLACE TNT

An individual is <u>never</u> a Failure. It is an event, plan, or relationship that may not be a success.

Acceptance is recognizing what is. It does not require liking, condoning or being happy about it.

Always hang on to the power of hope. You need hope in order to heal.

Appreciate achievement.

Balance and moderation are essentials for healthy growth and development.

Be a Fact Finder, not a Fault Finder.

Caring, compassion, communication, cooperation, and consistency are the "c's" that will positively see you through.

Do not judge or deny. Simply learn to identify.

Do not waste today on things you cannot control.

Each day brings new learning experiences and endless opportunities. Choose to make it positively work for you.

Each One is responsible for his/her own feelings, words, thoughts, beliefs, attitudes, actions, successes, and failures.

Each "put down" lowers a person's self-esteem.

Embrace enthusiasm.

Emotional energy is contagious. Be the one who fills your immediate environment with good cheer.

Everything requires time and energy. Energy spent <u>dwelling</u> on past painful thoughts is unproductive use of your time and energy.

Find something good in each day.

Focus on what <u>is</u> happening - instead of what <u>might</u> happen.

Focus on what you <u>can</u> do, instead of what you <u>can't</u> do.

Human beings are creatures of habit -- in what they think, say, and do. All habits are learned. No one is born with habits.

It is better to comfort than to confront.

It is okay to be full of awe by the overwhelming wonders of the world. It is not okay to be awfully overwhelmed.

Look forward to learning something new each day.

No two Individuals can agree on what is fair. It is a waste of time and energy to try to determine fairness.

Opt for optimism.

Patience means knowing it will happen and giving it time to happen.

Perfection is unattainable and unrealistic. Striving for perfection is an exercise in futility. It sets one up for failure. Eliminate the proverb "Practice makes perfect". Replace with "Practice makes better".

Prior planning prevents poor performance.

Regardless of your location, whether it is North, East, West, or South, seek positive exposure.

Recognize and appreciate your own importance and value.

Reduce the tendency to use the words "no", "not" or "never" before thinking things through.

Rewards are important motivators for habit change.

Responsibility for making things happen is strictly yours. It depends on what you choose to do. When you trust to luck, you attribute responsibility for success and achievement to an outside source.

Spend your time and energy seeking joy and satisfaction and there will be no room for anger and dissatisfaction.

Strive to be part of the solution, not part of the problem.

Successful outcomes are based upon good choices and good timing. Good timing requires realistic planning.

The shortest distance between identifying problems and reaching realistic solutions is keeping your eyes focused on specific facts, issues and circumstances.

Taking personal responsibility means not blaming anyone else for anything you are feeling or doing. It means setting a realistic goal and working towards achieving it.

Taking on more than one goal at a time, creates confusion.

The best time to express hurt feelings, is the moment it occurs-- before the pain turns to chronic anger.

The way to go to become the best that you can be, is from the inside-out.

The write way to say "no" to negative statements is to write "yes" statements.

The more you move forward, the more you distance yourself from the past.

The person who consistently comments on the way things "should" be, ignores the way things really are.

There is no future in the past.

To achieve efficiency, you must first identify and remedy the existing deficiency.

Unrealistic expectations set you up for disappointment and failure. Use your energy for what you can realistically do today.

What matters is what works well for you.

Whatever is more or less, is not balanced.

When you resist change, you miss new pathways for growth and challenge.

When you choose to accept, appreciate, and compliment, you cease to accuse, blame, and criticize.

When you take the angry words of others personally, you become emotionally involved and lose sight of your ability to focus on relevant issues.

When you cannot change a situation, you can change your outlook of the situation.

When you make peace with the painful past, you can then move on to a peaceful present.

When you come down with criticisms, you don't come up with suggestions.

When you come down with complaints, you don't come up with compliments.

With each passing moment, tomorrow becomes today.

You are the One who has won, when you recognize and appreciate that you are an important One.

Your Mind is a tool for you to use as you choose.

You cannot get ahead when you constantly look back.

Zero in to what is within.

Rx FOR LIFELONG PEP, HOPE, HEALTH AND HAPPINESS
A DAILY DOSE OF 8 B'S TO KEEP IN MIND

Be as busy as a buzzing bee using your 5 senses - sight, sound, smell, taste and touch – to learn something new each day.

Be the best you can be. Practice makes better.

Be your own best Pen Pal. Write more and stress less.

Be the 'I' you want to be. You are who you believe you are.

Be kind and good to your self. Love, honor, respect and protect your brain and body.

Be of good cheer.

Believe in your self and in your power to triumph over adversity. Self-confidence grows each time you overcome an exposure to adversity.

Be the one to share-a-smile with yourself and others.

BOTTOM LINE
A SHARED SMILE IS THE BEST GIFT ANYONE CAN GIVE OR GET.

A Daily 25 Minute, 5 step Bedtime Routine for Getting a Good Night's Sleep

Choosing to adopt, adapt, and apply this daily bedtime routine relieves emotional stress, physical tension and allows your mind and body to relax, rest comfortably and recharge itself with positive energy.

1. Spend 5 minutes writing about any angry or anxious concerns you are feeling. **When finished, tear up your comments. They are not to be kept or shared.**

2. Spend 5 minutes taking at least 5 deep breaths.

3. Spend 5 minutes briefly recording whatever you saw, heard, read or did that caused you to smile or laugh.

4. Spend 5 minutes increasing your smile mileage by doing tension-free smile doodling. Write rows and rows of a's, o's, e's, l's and fill them in with smiles – 2 dots and a curve.

5. Spend 5 minutes writing and reading PEP One-liners.

Take time to have fun. Keep smiling. Yes!!! Yes!!! Yes!!!

EVERY MINUTE SPENT

Every minute spent on worry is more than a minute lost
Because worry grows and festers at much too great a cost
Every minute spent on negativity insidiously destroys the soul
It causes sadness within your body and in time takes its toll
Every minute spent without thoughts of enthusiasm and hope
Makes it more difficult to function and ultimately to cope
What can we do to turn this negative cycle around
With proper strategies, a viable solution can be found

Take several deep breaths when you find there's need
Listen to your positive affirmations and then take heed
Count your blessings, even those that may be in disguise
Within minutes your mood will elevate and begin to rise
Enjoy the air, water and food that we all need to exist
But add to that a sprinkling of fun – try not to resist
Provide daily heartfelt gestures and aim to please
Good feelings will then come back to you with ease

Create a circle of love with hugs and words so kind
It will provide comfort and leave negativity behind
Smile at those you meet, and in the mirror, you as well
It will do wonders, making others and you feel just swell
Look toward nature and whatever comforts you choose
Put these strategies together as a daily cocktail to use
Try to solve the challenges you can, the best way you know how
Then life will take care of the others, allowing relaxation for now

Rita Kaufman

MOTIVATIONAL TEXT MESSAGES

Key Words To Keep In Mind

Words do matter. Every word – positive or negative- read, heard or spoken, can affect your heart rate, blood pressure and breathing in a fraction of a second.

AAA	Adopt, Adapt, Apply.
ATP	Activate The Positive.
BIYS	Believe In Your Self.
BOM	Be Open-Minded.
BYOH	Be Your Own Hero.
CFG	Compliments Feel Good.
CIA	Challenge Inaccurate Assumptions.
COC	Cut Out Comparisons
COS	Cut Out Sugar.
CCC	Calm, Cool, Connected.
CTSP	Compromise To Solve Problems.
CYM	Change Your Mindset.
DBCD	Deep Breathe – Calm Down.
DYB	Do Your Best.
EBC	Every Bite Counts.
EMM	Each Moment Matters.
ETM	Enjoy The Moment.
EYL	Enjoy Your Life.
FOCC	Focus On Complimentary Comments.
FOF	Focus On Facts
FOS	Focus On Specifics.
GCD	Give Compliments Daily.
HTS	Halt The Salt.
IBA	Imagine, Believe, Achieve.
IYC	It's Your Choice.
KDF	Knowledge Dispels Fear.
KMO	Keep Moving On.
KOS	Keep On Smiling.
LDA	Love Dispels Anger.
LFT	Live For Today.
LITM	Live In The Moment.
LLF	Live Life Fully.
LLL	Love, Learn, Laugh.

LLW	Live Life Wisely.
MBC	Moderation, Balance, Consistency.
MEC	Maintain Eye Contact.
MIH	Make It Happen.
MIR	Make "IT" Relevant.
MWD	Make Wise Decisions.
MYOS	Make Your Own Sunshine.
NYN	Nurture Your Nature.
OAU	Onward And Upward.
OSS	Organized Simple Schedules.
OFO	Opt For Optimism.
PAL	Patient Attentive Listener.
PEP	Positive Energy Power.
PMB	Practice Makes Better.
PSM	Portion Size Matters.
QYIQ	Quell Your Inner Qualms.
RYA	Recognize Your Achievements.
SAS	Share A Smile.
SITM	Stay In The Moment.
SPC	Support Positive Change.
STS	Strive, Thrive, Survive.
SYL	Simplify Your Life
TBA	Think, Believe, Achieve.
THT	Think Happy Thoughts.
TMT	Take "Me" Time.
TPM	Treasure Pleasurable Moments.
TTIN	The Time Is Now.
URU	You Are Unique.
VY	Value Yourself.
WDM	Words Do Matter.
WMSL	Write More, Stress Less.
WMWL	Write More, Weigh Less.
WSA	Write Stress Away.
WYSP	Wear Your Smile Proudly.
YAC	You Are Capable.
YIC	Yes I Can.

ROUTE 8 – THE FOOD/MOOD CONNECTION – THE CHEMICAL/ EMOTIONAL ENERGY CONNECTION

ESSENTIALS FOR A POSITIVELY ENERGIZED RELATIONSHIP WITH FOOD

THE STRESS AND SUGAR CONNECTION

SUBSTANCES THAT CAN CAUSE PHYSICAL AND EMOTIONAL DISORDERS

A FOOD PALETTE FOR YOUR PALATE

FOOD FOR THOUGHT

ESSENTIALS FOR A POSITIVELY ENERGIZED
RELATIONSHIP WITH FOOD

You are in charge of your feelings and your food choices. You control your emotional reactions -- how you respond to people, events, and situations. You control what will pass through your lips and enter your body. Your lips follow your orders. They open with your approval and remain closed until they get your approval.

Your Brain and Body need energy in order to function. Feelings provide emotional energy. Food provides chemical energy.

Food is made up of chemicals called nutrients. Nutrients are complex carbohydrates, proteins, essential fats, vitamins, and minerals. A daily consumption and combination of complex carbohydrates, proteins, essential fats, vitamins, minerals and water are the essential nutrients for meeting your unique chemical energy needs.

Complex Carbohydrates are converted into glucose – the chemical energy that is needed for the Brain and Nervous System. Glucose is needed to maintain a steady Blood Sugar Level. A fluctuating Blood Sugar Level adversely affects the functioning of the Brain and Nervous System and can contribute to aggressive, anti-social behavior.

Food sources for Complex Carbohydrates: barley, beans, buckwheat, corn, fresh fruits, leafy vegetables, legumes, natural whole grains, millet, oats, rye, wheat, nuts.

Protein is broken down into Amino Acids. Amino Acids are responsible for the growth, maintenance and repair of all your body cells –blood, bones, eyes, glands, heart, ligaments, lungs, muscles, nerves, organs, skin, teeth and tendons. Amino Acids produce the chemicals necessary for effective message transmission between your Brain and your Nervous System. Amino Acids strengthen the Immune System. One missing essential Amino Acid can create a Protein Deficiency, affect your energy level and lead to physical disorders. Every cell in your body contains and needs a continuous supply of Protein. Your body cells are constantly in need of repair and replacement. Your need for Protein is increased by exercise, stress and illness.

Food sources for Protein

Food of animal origin contain all the Amino Acids: lean meat, poultry, seafood, eggs, non-fat milk, cheese.

Vegetable sources of Protein contain vitamins, minerals, complex carbohydrates and fiber: beans, brown rice, grains, lentils, peas, plain non-fat yogurt, seeds, soybean products, tofu, unsalted raw nuts, whole grain cereals, wheat germ.

Essential Fatty Acids maintain the Cardio-Vascular, Immune and Nervous Systems, distribute fat soluble vitamins A,D,E,K throughout the body and insulate the nerves. The billions of nerve cells in the Brain need a daily dose of Essential Fatty Acids to function effectively.

Food sources for Essential Fatty Acids: avocados, nuts, seeds, soybeans, wheat germ, cold water fish oils –mackerel, salmon, sardines, vegetable oils – canola, olive, safflower, sesame.

VITAMINS A, B-COMPLEX, C, D AND E ARE ANTI-STRESS NUTRIENTS THAT ENHANCE THE IMMUNE SYSTEM, COMBAT STRESS AND KEEP EVERY BODY CELL OPTIMALLY ENERGIZED.

Vitamin A (Beta Carotene) stimulates the Immune System to protect the body against infection, builds resistance to respiratory infections, protects the body against environmental pollution, repairs and maintains the health of the skin, eyes and hair. Vitamin A promotes the growth of strong bones, teeth and gums.

Food Sources for Vitamin A

Green, yellow and orange fruits and vegetables, apricots, asparagus, broccoli, cantaloupe, carrots, mangoes, papaya, peaches, spinach, yellow squash, sweet potatoes, pumpkin, eggs, milk.

Vitamin B-complex builds the cell's immunity to infection, stabilizes the Nervous System by decreasing irritability and improving concentration, memory and mood. Vitamin B-complex helps to form the healthy red blood cells that deliver oxygen to the body and converts carbohydrates into glucose- the chemical energy for the brain and nerves.

Food sources for Vitamin B-complex:

brown rice, eggs, fish, poultry, lean meat, cheese, green leafy vegetables, beans, broccoli, cabbage, carrots, peas, spinach, pumpkin, sesame, sunflower seeds, nuts, soybeans, wheat germ, whole grains, oatmeal, wheat bran, yogurt.

Vitamin C increases the white blood cell activity, preventing viral and bacterial infections, aids in the growth and repair of body tissues and promotes the healing of wounds.

Food sources for Vitamin C:

green leafy vegetables, berries, cantaloupe, broccoli, cauliflower, grapefruit, honeydew, kiwi, lemons, mangoes, papaya, potatoes, strawberries, tangerines, tomatoes, watermelon.

Vitamin D stimulates the Immune System, improves muscular function, helps to maintain strong bones and reduce the risk of bone disease and fractures.
Food sources for Vitamin D:
salmon, sardines, shrimp, eggs, fortified milk.

Vitamin E improves blood circulation, repairs body tissues and promotes healing.
Food sources for Vitamin E:
avocado, brown rice, dark green leafy vegetables, spinach, broccoli, brussels sprouts, eggs, nuts, seeds, wheat germ, whole grain cereals, peanut butter, vegetable oils, soybeans.

THE ANTI-STRESS MINERALS – CALCIUM, MAGNESIUM, SELENIUM AND ZINC- ARE ESSENTIAL FOR NERVE, MUSCLE AND NORMAL CELL ACTIVITY.

Calcium, a major bone building mineral, plays an important role in the formation and maintenance of strong, healthy bones and teeth, aids in muscle growth, alleviates tension, irritability and insomnia and relaxes the nerves.
Food sources for Calcium are:
low fat milk, low fat cheeses, low fat yogurt, dried beans, green vegetables, peanuts, sardines, salmon, sunflower seeds, soybeans.

Magnesium - necessary for Calcium and Vitamin C metabolism- improves the Cardio-Vascular System, relieves indigestion and improves mood.
Food sources for Magnesium are:
almonds, apples, apricots, corn, dark green vegetables, figs, grapefruit, lemons, nuts, seeds.

Selenium works with Vitamin E and improves the functioning of the Heart and Lungs.
Food sources for Selenium are:
bran, broccoli, onions, tomatoes, tuna, wheat germ.

Zinc plays a vital role in regulating the Immune System, promotes growth, mental alertness and heals wounds.

Food sources for Zinc are:

eggs, lamb chops, non-fat dry milk, pumpkin seeds, wheat germ.

THE STRESS AND SUGAR CONNECTION

Our Sympathetic Nervous System automatically responds to emotional stress - feelings of anger, fear, sadness, anxiety and worry. Digestion, heart, blood pressure and breathing are affected. Stress hormones are released, blood is diverted away from the digestive system to the musculature and the digestive system is prevented from performing its normal function. Emotional stress is known to intensify cravings for sugar.

EXCLUDE REFINED SIMPLE SUGAR FROM YOUR DAILY FOOD PLAN.

Refined simple sugar creates a short-lived, quick burst of energy followed by a fast fall in energy level. Simple sugar over-stimulates the pancreas, causing it to overreact. Simple sugar causes the adrenal glands to over-secrete adrenaline. Simple sugar decreases the oxygen supply to body tissues and can contribute to fatigue, depression, hyperactivity, obesity and inability to concentrate.

Sugar in processed foods can cause extreme fluctuations in blood sugar level. Sugar is found in almost all processed foods—soda, fruit drinks, frozen dinners, breads, cereals, cakes, cookies, canned foods, candy bars, pies, chewing gum, toothpaste and medicines.

Sugar by any other name is still simply Simple Sugar:

brown sugar (table sugar with molasses coating), corn syrup, dextrose, glucose, honey, lactose (milk sugar), maltose, maple sugar, molasses, sucrose (table sugar), fructose (fruit sugar from fruits, juices,--the only simple sugar that provides a slower, steady supply of blood sugar suitable for diabetics).

To diminish cravings for sugar, consume more whole grains, sweet potatoes, apples, apricots and raisins. Munch on crunchy stress relieving foods: pop corn, raw vegetables, carrots, graham crackers, rice cakes and bran cereal. Use desserts sweetened with barley malt, or rice syrup. Cultivate a taste for sour foods: unsweetened grapefruit and lemonade.

BOTTOM LINE

READ LABELS ON ALL PACKAGED FOODS IN ORDER TO MAKE HEALTHY CHOICES. IF IN DOUBT, LEAVE IT OUT.

SUBSTANCES THAT CAN CAUSE PHYSICAL AND EMOTIONAL DISORDERS

Alcohol depletes the body of B vitamins, Calcium, Magnesium and Zinc, impairs muscle coordination, weakens the Immune System and intensifies feelings of anxiety, depression and fatigue.

Caffeine in coffee, tea, colas, chocolate, energy drinks, diet pills and headache remedies, depletes the body of B vitamins, potassium and zinc, restricts the blood flow to the Brain, contributes to anxiety, fatigue, dizziness, headaches, insomnia, irritability, memory problems, nervousness and shakiness. Caffeine can cause heart irregularities and a rise in Blood Pressure.

Nicotine depletes the body of Vitamins B and C and Calcium, elevates Blood Pressure, causes constriction of the arterial blood vessels in the heart, coughs, headaches, mood swings and damages muscle and nerve metabolism.

Salt contributes to High Blood Pressure and overworked Kidneys, causes water retention (excessive fluid build-up in the body tissues) and interferes with the blood's ability to transport metabolic waste for excretion. Salt interferes with the blood's ability to carry nutrients and oxygen to all the body cells.

Food allergies stress the Immune System so that the body becomes vulnerable to disease. Food allergies can contribute to hypertension, tension headaches, anxiety attacks and an increase in heartbeats in adults and hyperactivity in children. Highly allergenic foods are: cereal, citrus fruits, chocolate, dairy products, eggs, poultry, red meat, shellfish, soybeans, strawberries, wheat, corn, barley, rye, oats, nuts, foods containing yeast. Daily consumption of a favorite food is often responsible for allergies. Rotation of foods is the best protection against allergies.

BE AN IDEAL FOOD ENERGY SELECTOR

The purpose of food is to supply your body with the chemicals and energy it needs for building cells and keeping your body systems working.
Become aware of the relationship between food and color energy. Recognize your daily energy needs. Use the Food Palette to select the foods that will supply your body needs with the necessary energies for daily optimum functioning.

A FOOD PALETTE FOR YOUR PALATE

Red Foods, rich in all B Vitamins, provide strong vitalizing physical energy.

Orange Foods, rich in Vitamins A, B, C, stimulate physical vitality and a feeling of Well-Being.

Yellow Foods, rich in Vitamins A, C, stimulate the metabolism.

Green Foods, rich in Vitamin C and Minerals, stimulate the nerves, relax and refresh the body.

Blue and Purple Foods calm the emotions.

Red Foods -- beets, tomatoes, radishes, red cabbage, red beans, dark red cherries, red currants, red plums, red grapes, raspberries, strawberries, watermelon, apples.

Orange Foods -- carrots, sweet potatoes, squash, pumpkins, peaches, apricots, cantaloupes, oranges, tangerines, nectarines, mangoes, papaya, persimmons, eggs, cheese.

Yellow Foods -- peppers, corn, yellow squash, parsnips, bananas, pineapple, lemons, grapefruit, figs, peaches, honeydew, melons, eggs, butter, yellow cheese, mustard.

Green Foods -- green beans, green peas, spinach, asparagus, cabbage, zucchini, green peppers, broccoli, cucumbers, avocado, green celery, raw green salads, parsley, olives.

Blue Foods -- blueberries, blue plums.

Purple Foods -- purple broccoli, eggplant, purple cabbage, prunes.

Timing and your feelings are significant factors that affect your body chemistry balance. The feelings that you experience at the time you eat your food, can positively or negatively modify the food's effect on your body chemistry.

For sustained optimum energy, select red, orange, yellow foods for your breakfast.

For a relaxed Nervous System, select green vegetables and salads as part of your evening meal. A relaxed Nervous System prepares your body for restful sleep -- the time needed for internal repair of cells and tissues in order to achieve renewed energy in the morning.

BOTTOM LINE

WHAT YOU EAT DETERMINES HOW WELL YOU FEEL, THINK, AND PERFORM!!!

YOUR VEGGIE PALS

We're your veggie pals found in your favorite store
Have us for breakfast, lunch and for dinner, some more
We're here to help you feel energized and snappy
In tip-top shape, cheery, positive and happy

We come in many colors, oh, so bright
We pack a wallop with each bite
Add dressing or spice, but just a sprinkle
We'll keep you healthy without a wrinkle

Eat us raw, in salad, soup or stew
We're your pals – we'll do great things for you
Place us generously upon your plate
We'll help to make your meal first rate

Share us with friends and family tonight
For parties and celebrations we fit just right
Choose your dish and prepare us in any way
We'll serve you well throughout each day

Rita Kaufman

SOUP, SALAD AND ...

A friend told me of a restaurant famous for salad and soup
He said, "It's great! Go and enjoy – be in the loop"
I opened the door and said, "What a great meal I'll make"
There are two long aisles of salad with everything to take

I took a plate and started from the beginning
And slowly a salad masterpiece I was creating
With my salad on the table to the soup aisle I went
I counted seven varieties and a happy signal was sent

Healthy soup and salad - two wonderful choices for sure
But I noticed delicious breads, muffins and much more
What happened to just the soup and salad, I thought
But into the other treats my excited eyes soon bought

I tried to resist, but the temptation was strong
It's clear that in this section I didn't belong
Okay, I did it – it's over - I'll be better next time
On that, for sure, you can bet more than a dime

Rita Kaufman

FOOD FOR THOUGHT

Choose foods that will provide optimum chemical energy, boost your Immune System and reduce your emotional stress. A chemically well-balanced nutritional program includes fresh fruits and vegetables, grains, beans, complex carbohydrates, and proteins. Several small meals throughout the day provides for a balanced blood sugar level. Breakfast is the most important meal of the day. Your memory and blood sugar level are affected when you skip breakfast.

ADOPT AND ADAPT THE 8-STEP PEP PLAN FOR VIM, VIGOR AND VITALITY.

1. Eliminate second helpings of any food.
2. Use smaller size plates and utensils for smaller size servings.
3. Eat slowly and be mindful of what you eat.
4. Stay out of the kitchen after 8 or 9 PM.
5. Prepare shopping lists ahead of time to avoid buying on impulse. Be sure to have stress-free snacks readily available to offset any sugar cravings.
6. Do not shop when you are hungry.
7. Prepare a PEP Journal (Pleasurably Engaged Plans)- positive action to keep your brain and body busy with activities you enjoy doing indoors and outside–hobbies, reading, writing, listening to music, gardening, volunteering, yoga. It's time to have fun. It's time to seek new interests.
8. Moderate walking exercise begins when doing your food shopping. Focus on the foods in the outer aisles where you are likely to find fruits, vegetables, dairy and grains.

BOTTOM LINE

YOU ARE WHAT YOU EAT!!!
MODERATION, BALANCE AND A STABLE BLOOD SUGAR LEVEL ARE THE KEYS TO FEELING GOOD FROM HEAD TO TOE!!!

FOOD, GLORIOUS FOOD – BUT WAY TOO MUCH

Last night we ate and partied, as we ate our dinner out
We consumed way too much – of that there is no doubt

We were many friends together at the table with our guys
Laughing, joking, reminiscing – the evening held such highs

The evening began about seven-thirty and continued until late
The dishes kept coming, one after the other – we sat and we ate

The night was an orgy in eating – it was hard to say "no"
But we all were hoping that our stomachs would not grow

The food was fried, fattening, too rich and laden with sauce
It was hard to make healthy choices and be our own good boss

The dishes tasted great, but by health standards, were not ideal
And now it's the next morning and the taste of guilt we feel

There were few appropriate choices to make, and so we made
none
But emotionally, the results took away some of last night's fun

Now we have to undo the damage our eating did create
And somehow get rid of all this unwanted, extra weight

Rita Kaufman

FOOD IS NOT THE ANSWER

A food challenge can be a daily thing
Distract with a hobby - dance or sing

Relax or meditate to keep your body stress-free
It's such a healthy and energizing way to be

Put feelings and thoughts on paper each day
Write them down to send negativity away

Exercise and eat right for optimal weight
Both serve to help you feel first rate

Solving problems can be hard to do
But food is not the solution for you

Solve your difficult issues in another way
Separate those from food choices made today

Take baby steps; be encouraged and proud of these
And then hour by hour, each day will go with ease

Rita Kaufman

ROUTE 9 – THE COLOR CONNECTION TO YOUR MOOD, CLOTHES AND ENVIRONMENT

THE COLOR VISUAL CONNECTION TO YOUR MOOD

THE CONNECTION BETWEEN YOUR EMOTIONAL NEEDS AND THE COLORS YOU CHOOSE
TO WEAR

THE IMPACT OF COLOR ENERGY ON YOUR BODY CHEMISTRY

THE COLOR/MOOD CONNECTION IN YOUR SURROUNDINGS

COLOR – The Visual Energy Connection to Your Mood

Color is a stimulant and can affect your energy level. Each person responds emotionally and physically to color stimulation. Your response to the color that you see is related to your past experiences, meaningful associations, and how you are physically and emotionally feeling at the time. Your emotional and physical state constantly fluctuates and your response to color fluctuates as well.

HOW DO COLORS AFFECT YOU?

Do you frown when you see brown?

Do you feel mellow when you wear yellow?

What do you say when you see gray?

Do you feel light and bright, when you wear white?

Do you like being seen when you wear green?

When buying clothes, do you leave anything black on the rack?

Are your worries shed, when you wear red?

Is blue just right for you?

Do you blink as others wink when you wear pink?

THE CONNECTION BETWEEN YOUR EMOTIONAL NEEDS AND THE COLORS YOU CHOOSE TO WEAR

Use the power of color energy to satisfy your daily emotional needs, give you a sense of well- being and answer the question "What color shall I wear?"

Do you need to feel calm, relaxed, serene, secure?

    Select Green, Light Blue, Turquoise.

Do you need to feel optimistic and cheerful?

    Select Yellow, Peach, Orange.

Do you need to feel safe and secure?

    Select Brown.

Do you feel emotionally fatigued?

    Select Grey.

IMPORTANT TO NOTE:

Avoid the severity of wearing only one solid color.

Red is the strongest color stimulant. Over exposure to Red can contribute to emotional stress and physical tension. Red is not recommended for highly excitable Individuals.

Use accessories -- jewelry, belts, scarves, ties, hats, shoes -- to diffuse the intensity of a color.

Use cool colors to neutralize the intensity of warm colors.

    Green and Turquoise neutralize Red and Brown.

    Blue neutralizes Orange.

    Purple neutralizes Yellow.

    Introduce accents of White, Black, or Grey.

THE IMPACT OF COLOR ENERGY ON YOUR BODY CHEMISTRY

Color energy affects the chemistry of all your Body Systems.

Warm colors are stronger stimulants than cool colors.

Red Color Energy produces the strongest intensity of stimulation to your Sympathetic Nervous System and speeds up your metabolism, raises your blood pressure, pulse rate, heart action, body heat, and increases your vitality.

Pink Color Energy produces a moderate degree of stimulation to your Sympathetic Nervous System and increases the blood supply to your Brain, and relaxes your mental tensions.

Orange Color Energy stimulates your blood circulation and your appetite and increases your physical and mental vitality.

Yellow Color Energy activates your body functions and stimulates your muscles and nerves.

Green Color Energy stimulates your Parasympathetic Nervous System, lowers your blood pressure, and relieves your muscle and nerve tension.

Turquoise Color Energy relieves your stress and tension.

Light Blue Color Energy produces a pacifying effect on your Parasympathetic Nervous System, slows down your Body Metabolism, lowers your blood pressure, pulse rate, heart action, body heat, and reduces your nervous tension.

Purple Color Energy lowers your blood pressure and calms your nerves.

THE COLOR/MOOD CONNECTION IN YOUR SURROUNDINGS

Warm colors -- Red, Yellow, Orange, -- create a warm atmosphere.

Red fosters excitement, high spirited physical activity, inhibits rest, relaxation, and concentration.

Yellow radiates optimism, encourages lively conversation, stimulates mental and creative activity.

Cool colors -- Green, Blue, Purple – create a cool atmosphere, a feeling of spaciousness, and encourage rest and relaxation.
Tones of Blue and Green reduce hyperactivity, encourage concentration, and are ideal peaceful settings for sedentary activities.
Violet provides an atmosphere for creative, imaginative self- expression.

Dark, drab colors lower morale, increase inhibitions.

All white in a room fosters loneliness.

Light Pink, Peach, Beiges, increase feelings of emotional support and security, decrease depression and loneliness.

Gray is restful.

ROUTE 10 – A COLLECTION OF WISE WORDS TO KEEP IN MIND

A COLLECTION OF WISE WORDS TO KEEP IN MIND

Flowing water never goes bad.

    Chinese proverb

Fall seven times, stand up eight.

    Japanese proverb

The closer you stand to the lighthouse, the darker it gets.

    Japanese proverb

There is always a piece of fortune in misfortune.

    Japanese proverb

The biggest room in the world is the room for improvement.

    Japanese proverb

Fortune comes to those who smile.

    Japanese proverb

One joy scatters a hundred griefs.

    Chinese proverb

Nonviolence requires much more courage than violence.

    Mahatma Gandhi

To be wronged is nothing unless you continue to remember it.

    Confucius

If everyday is an awakening, you will never grow old. You will just keep growing.

    Gail Sheehy

Fear is that little darkroom where negatives are developed.

    Michael Pritchard

The time is always right to do what is right.

    Martin Luther King, Jr.

A single rose can be my garden, a single friend my world.

    Lee Buscaglia

Laughter is the joyous, universal evergreen of life.

    Abraham Lincoln

I have found that most people are about as happy as they make up their minds to be.

    Abraham Lincoln

Things turn out best for the people who make the best out of the way things turn out.   Art Linkletter.

Kind words can be short and easy to speak but their echoes are truly endless.

    Mother Teresa

Peace starts with a smile.

Mother Teresa

A smile is the universal welcome.

Max Eastman

A warm smile is the universal language of kindness.

William Arthur Ward

All people smile in the same language.

Proverb

A smile is happiness right under your nose.

Tom Watson

He who smiles rather than rages is always the stronger.

Japanese proverb

You cannot put out fires with flames.

Turkish proverb

Love is the master key which opens the gates of happiness.

Oliver Wendell Holmes, Sr.

One word frees us all the weight and pain of life. That word is love.

Sophocles

Education is the best provision for the journey to old age.

Aristotle (384-322 B.C.)

We are formed and molded by our thoughts.

Buddha

What we think, we become.

Buddha

Joy is not in things. It is in us.

Benjamin Franklin

Faith is like electricity. You can't see it but you can see the light.

Anonymous

A dream doesn't become a reality through magic; it takes sweat, determination and hard work.

Colin Powell

The only place you find success before work, is in the dictionary.

Mary V. Smith

Most of the things worth doing in the world had been declared impossible before they were done.

Louis Brandeis

There are 2 days about which nobody should ever worry and these are "yesterday" and "tomorrow".

Robert J. Burdett

Positive anything is better than negative nothing.

    Elbert Hubbard

Worry often gives a small thing a big shadow.

    Swedish saying

Live the life you imagined.

    Henry David Thoreau

Go confidently in the direction of your dream.

    Henry David Thoreau

Be the change you wish to see in the world.

    Mahatma Gandhi

Colors fade, temples crumble, empires fall but wise words endure.

    Edward Thorndike

ROUTE 11 – WORD-GAME ACTIVITY TO POSITIVELY ACTIVATE THE BRAIN

WORD SEARCH

WHAT'S IN A NAME

WORD SEARCH

What word begins and ends with the letter "s", has 34 letters and means "good"?
The word appears in a song in "Mary Poppins".

Answer:
SUPERCALIFRAGILISTICEXPIALIDOCIOUS

How many words of 3, 4, 5 or more letters are hidden within this one word? Don't
be surprised if you can find more than 100 words in each category.

Helpful clues to increase your word search score
Look for consonants to build rhyming families

    dill, drill, fill, frill, gill, grill, pill, spill, still, till

    case, grace, lace, pace, race, ace

Use suffix endings

Suffixes are letters that are added to the end of a word.

An adjective + suffix "er"	tall+ er= taller
A verb + suffix "ed"	roar+ed= roared
A verb+ suffix "s"	roar+s=roars
A noun+suffix "s"	fact+s=facts
A noun+suffix "ful" becomes an adjective	success+ful=successful
A noun+ suffix "less" becomes an adjective	fear+less=fearless

Endless Sources for a daily dose of Word Search – texts from newspapers,
magazines, books, the dictionary.

Homophones - words that have the same sound but are different in spelling and
meaning - can serve to increase your word search score.

ad - add	leak - leek	nay - neigh
ail - ale	leased - least	need - knead
air - heir	lesson - lessen	new - knew
aisle - isle	lie - lye	night-knight
all - awl	links - lynx	nit - knit
aloud - allowed	loan - lone	no - know
altar - alter	maid - made	none - nun

ant - aunt	mail - male	nose - knows	
arc - ark	main - mane	not - knot	
ate - eight	mall - maul	ode - owed	
aural - oral	manner - manor	oar - ore	
aye - eye - I	marshall - martial	our - hour	
dear - deer	meddle - medal	tacks - tax	
dents - dense	mince - mints	tale - tail	
dew - do - due	minds - mines	taught - taut	
die - dye	miner - minor	tea - tee	
doe - dough	mite - might	team - teem	
earn - urn	mode - mowed	tear - tier	
gait - gate	morn - mourn	tense - tents	
grate - great	morning - mourning	their - their	
groan - grown	naval - navel	thyme - time	
lead - led	thrown - throne	toe-tow	
tide - tied	threw-through	toad-towed	
too - to - two			

Instantly double your word search score with words that form different words when they are read and written backwards.

bat	tab	slap	pals
but	tub	stab	bats
draw	ward	star	rats
keep	peek	step	pets
live	evil	stop	pots
mood	doom	strap	parts
net	ten	stun	nuts
no	on	tap	pat
not	ton	tar	rat
now	won	teem	meet
pan	nap	tip	pit
par	rap	top	pot
ram	mar	trap	part
reed	deer	was	saw
reward	drawer	wed	dew

WHAT'S IN A NAME?

How many words are hidden within the letters of your name?

Write your First, Middle and Last Name.

List all the little words you can form from the letters in your name.

Write one or more messages using as many of these words as possible.

Exchange names with another person. Repeat the activity.

Who discovered more words?

Who wrote more messages?

Expand your fun activity by randomly selecting names of those you know and don't know.

I found 124 words in Hillary Rodham Clinton's name. Can you top that?

Helpful Clue

Look for rhyming words to quickly increase your word list.

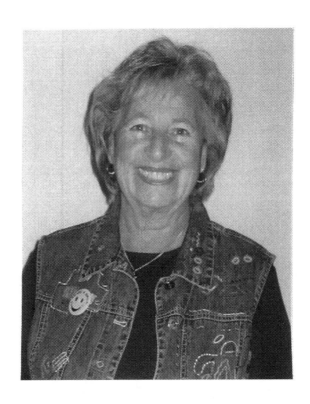

ABOUT RITA KAUFMAN

Rita Kaufman is a graduate of Parsons School of Design and New York University. She holds a Bachelor of Science degree from N.Y.U. and a Master of Science degree from Brooklyn College. She is a retired teacher with more than thirty years experience teaching Pre-kindergarten through Grade one and Junior-high school art. She authored three teacher manuals entitled <u>A Joyful Journey to Miles of Smiles</u>. The first was written as a result of a Pilot Program and is geared to Grades 3-6. The second is for Grades Pre K-Grade 2 and the third for children ages three to five. She taught art classes at Silver Gull Club, Surf Club and the Kings Bay Y. Since retirement, she presents workshops for teachers and works with children in the classroom.

Her poems were written because of the inspiration of Edith Namm while taking her classes at Brooklyn College. They were a direct result of self-discovery and her desire to adopt and apply the principles learned from Mrs. Namm.

Her family, Neil, Paul, Rhona, Jenna, Michael, Alyssa, Bryan, Matt and David bring her much joy and miles of smiles!

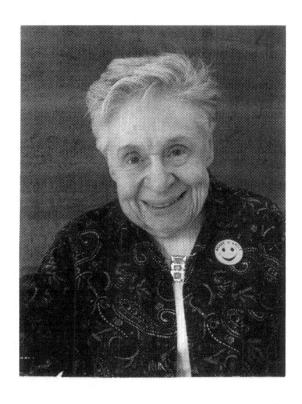

ABOUT EDITH NAMM

Counselor and Specialized Handwriting Analyst, holding a Master's Degree in Guidance from New York University and Certification as a Specialized Graphoanalyst from the Institute of Graphological Science, Texas University, Dallas, Texas.

25 years of experience as a Guidance Counselor, over 20 years of experience as a Specialized Handwriting Analyst.

Honored as "The Outstanding Counselor" in District 21, Brooklyn, N.Y. in 1986.

A thyroid, breast, colon, liver cancer survivor, who has authored six books on stress management and is dedicated to sharing safe, simple self-help techniques that can positively energize one's brain and body.

On the IRPE (Institute for Retirees in Pursuit of Education) faculty at Brooklyn College teaching a course on stress management, *A Joyful Journey to Miles of Smiles.*. Teaching a teleconference course, *The Write Way To a Positively Energized Brain and Body*, on Dorot's University Without Walls-To Your Health Program.

Founder of Share-a-Smile Ambassadors, whose mission is:

To activate school, home and community Share-a-Smile Projects that effectively relieve emotional stress, raise self-esteem, promote positive social interaction, establish healthy relationships and increase one's positive energy power regardless of age, gender or economic background.

TO CHANGE THE WORLD, ONE SMILE AT A TIME.

Producer of *The Lyrical Way to Miles of Smiles*

A CD that can empower children to reduce emotional stress and physical tension, and activate the thoughts that lead to a positive self-image, a positive attitude, socially acceptable behavior and healthy relationships.

Producer of *Loving Lullabies – The Lyrical Way to Miles of Smiles for Everyone*

A CD collection of musical messages that encourage peaceful rest, pleasant dreams, and provide the comfort, security, reassurance, and love that is essential for a child's healthy emotional development.

Developer and Producer of *The Write Way to a Positively Energized Brain and Body.*

An on-line course to introduce participants to PEP (Positive Energy Power) Aerobics – safe, simple, self-help strategies that positively energize the brain and body and empower one to be healthy and happy from sunrise to sunset.

Edith Namm believes that being married to Larry for 62 years, a mother to Diane and Dale and Nana to Kathryn, Michael, Justin and Vanessa has positively enriched her journey to miles of Smiles and Positive Energy Power.

BOOKS WRITTEN BY EDITH NAMM, M.A., C.S.G.

A Joyful Journey to Positive Parenting

A comprehensive approach and guide to miles of smiles featuring:
PEP (Positive Energy Power) Aerobics –specialized handwriting exercises designed to empower a parent and child to feel confident, experience a positive state of well-being and effectively cope with the stress of daily living.
The ABC's for positive parenting/child relationships and effective communication in a safe, nurturing home environment.
The color energy connection to mood, food, clothes and environment.

Learning to See What A Child's Handwriting Shows and Tells

A resource manual that teaches educators, counselors and psychologists how to identify fear, depression and anger in a child's handwriting and provides specialized handwriting exercises that show children how to counteract those feelings and achieve a positive state of well-being.

The Write Way to Go From Stress to Serenity

A stress-management manual, dedicated to all those whose lives are touched by Cancer, offers specialized handwriting exercises that are designed to reduce emotional stress and increase feelings of well-being.

The Winning Ways to Relieve Stress and Increase Positive Energy Power (PEP)

A stress-management guide that illustrates how food, color and specialized handwriting exercises can empower a writer to feel confident, self-fulfilled and achieve a positive outlook on life.

The Write Way to Positive Parenting

A stress management manual that explains how writing can empower a parent and child to feel confident and successfully cope with daily stress.

Rhyming Riddles and Tons of Tongue Twisters for Miles of Smiles
Dedicated to children of all ages, the book celebrates the healing power of smiles and laughter to relieve stress and positively energize the mind, body, and spirit.